AFIB DIET COOKBOOK

A Beginners and Seniors Guide with Heart-Healthy Meal Plans and Diet Recipes with Pictures

Jim Amos

TABLE OF CONTENT

INTRODUCTION

Welcome to the "Afib Diet Cookbook," your essential guide to living well and eating right while managing atrial fibrillation. If you or a loved one has been diagnosed with Afib, you understand the challenges it brings to everyday life. This book is here to help you navigate those challenges with delicious, heart-healthy recipes and expert dietary advice.

Atrial fibrillation, commonly known as Afib, is a heart condition that causes irregular and often rapid heartbeats. This can lead to blood clots, stroke, heart failure, and other heart-related complications. Managing Afib requires a comprehensive approach, including medication, lifestyle changes, and crucially, a heart-healthy diet.

Eating well when you have Afib doesn't mean sacrificing flavor or enjoyment. The recipes in this cookbook are designed to support heart health without compromising on taste. We've crafted meals that are rich in essential nutrients, low in sodium and unhealthy fats, and full of vibrant flavors. From hearty breakfasts and satisfying lunches to delicious dinners and tempting desserts, every recipe is crafted with your well-being in mind.

But this book is more than just a collection of recipes. It's a roadmap to a healthier lifestyle. You'll find tips on choosing the right ingredients, advice on portion control, and guidance on avoiding foods that can trigger Afib episodes. We've included practical strategies to help you make heart-smart choices whether you're cooking at home, dining out, or planning meals for a busy week.

The "**Afib Diet Cookbook**" is grounded in the latest scientific research and dietary recommendations for managing atrial fibrillation. We've worked with nutritionists, cardiologists, and culinary experts to bring you a resource that is both informative and enjoyable to use. Our goal is to empower you with the knowledge and tools to take control of your health through mindful eating.

Embark on this culinary journey to better health, where every meal is an opportunity to nourish your body and support your heart. Whether you're newly diagnosed with Afib or looking for fresh, nutritious ideas to enhance your existing diet, this cookbook will be your trusted companion in the kitchen.

Here's to a healthier heart and a happier life. Enjoy the journey!

CHAPTER ONE

WHAT IS ATRIAL FIBRILLATION?

Atrial Fibrillation is a type of irregular heartbeat, or arrhythmia, that affects millions of people worldwide.

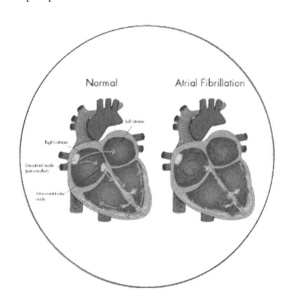

It occurs when the electrical signals in your heart's upper chambers (the atria) become chaotic, causing the heart to beat irregularly and often rapidly. Instead of a smooth, coordinated contraction, the atria quiver, which can lead to a variety of symptoms and potential complications.

You might be wondering, "How does this actually feel?" Well, symptoms can vary widely. Some people experience palpitations, which feel like a fluttering or racing heart. Others might have shortness of breath, fatigue, dizziness, or even chest pain. And here's the tricky part: some folks have no symptoms at all and only discover they have AFib during a routine check-up.

Now, why should we be concerned about AFib? The irregular beating of the heart can lead to poor blood flow, and when blood doesn't flow properly, it can pool and form clots. These clots can travel to the brain, causing a stroke, which is one of the most serious complications of AFib. In fact, people with AFib are five times more likely to have a stroke compared to those without the condition. Other complications can include heart failure, where the heart can't pump blood effectively, and other cardiovascular problems.

The good news is that with proper management, including dietary changes, medication, and lifestyle modifications, you can significantly reduce the risks associated with AFib. That's where this cookbook comes in! We'll explore delicious, heart-healthy recipes that can help you manage your condition and live a healthier, happier life.

History and Causes of Atrial Fibrillation

Let's take a step back and look at the history and causes of AFib. Understanding where it comes from can help us appreciate the importance of managing it.

A Brief History

AFib isn't a new condition; it's been around for centuries. Early descriptions of irregular heartbeats can be traced back to ancient Greek and Chinese medical texts. However, it wasn't until the 20th century that medical advancements allowed for a deeper understanding of the condition. In the early 1900s, with the invention of the electrocardiogram (ECG or EKG), doctors could visually capture and study the heart's electrical activity, paving the way for diagnosing AFib accurately.

Understanding the Causes

AFib can be caused by a variety of factors, and often it's a combination of several elements. Here are some common causes:

- Heart-Related Conditions: High Blood Pressure (Hypertension): This is one of the leading causes. Over time, high blood pressure can cause the heart's muscle tissue to thicken and become stiff, disrupting the normal electrical signals.

- Heart Disease: Conditions such as coronary artery disease, heart valve issues, and heart failure can increase the risk of developing AFib.

- Congenital Heart Defects: Some people are born with heart abnormalities that can predispose them to AFib.

Non-Heart-Related Factors

- Age: The risk of AFib increases as we get older. It's more common in people over 60, but it can occur at any age.

- Thyroid Problems: Both hyperthyroidism (overactive thyroid) and hypothyroidism (underactive thyroid) can contribute to the development of AFib.

- Sleep Apnea: This condition, characterized by interrupted breathing during sleep, is a significant risk factor for AFib.

- Chronic Conditions: Diabetes, chronic kidney disease, and obesity are all associated with a higher risk of AFib.

Benefits of an AFib Diet for Beginners

Adopting an AFib-friendly diet can be a game-changer in managing this condition. Not only does it help reduce the symptoms, but it also addresses the underlying risk factors that contribute to AFib. Here are five benefits of following an AFib diet for beginners:

- **Heart Health Optimization:** A well-planned AFib diet emphasizes heart-healthy foods that are low in unhealthy fats and rich in essential nutrients. This includes plenty of fruits, vegetables, whole grains, lean proteins, and healthy fats like those found in nuts and fish. These foods help maintain a healthy weight, reduce blood pressure, and lower cholesterol levels—all crucial factors in managing AFib.

For instance, incorporating omega-3 fatty acids from fatty fish such as salmon or plant sources like flaxseeds and walnuts can help reduce inflammation and improve heart rhythm stability. Additionally, antioxidants found in colorful fruits and vegetables protect the heart by neutralizing harmful free radicals.

- **Blood Pressure Regulation:** High blood pressure is a significant risk factor for AFib, and diet plays a crucial role in controlling it. By reducing the intake of sodium and increasing potassium-rich foods, you can help maintain healthy blood pressure levels. Foods like bananas, sweet potatoes, spinach, and avocados are excellent sources of potassium.

Moreover, a diet low in processed foods and rich in whole, unprocessed ingredients naturally reduces sodium intake. Herbs and spices can be used to flavor food without the need for excess salt, making meals both healthy and delicious.

- **Weight Management** Excess weight is closely linked to the development and worsening of AFib. An AFib diet focuses on nutrient-dense, low-calorie foods that help with weight management. By prioritizing vegetables, fruits, lean proteins, and whole grains, you can achieve a healthy weight, which in turn reduces the strain on your heart and improves your overall cardiovascular health.

Intermittent fasting or mindful eating practices can also be incorporated into your

9

diet plan to prevent overeating and promote better weight control. These strategies encourage a balanced approach to eating, helping you stay on track with your dietary goals.

- Reduced Inflammation: Chronic inflammation is a contributing factor to many heart diseases, including AFib. Anti-inflammatory foods such as leafy greens, berries, nuts, and fatty fish are staples in an AFib diet. These foods contain bioactive compounds like polyphenols, flavonoids, and omega-3 fatty acids that help combat inflammation and support heart health.

For example, consuming a daily serving of berries like blueberries or strawberries provides a significant dose of antioxidants and vitamins that reduce oxidative stress and inflammation. Similarly, incorporating green leafy vegetables into meals ensures a steady supply of essential nutrients that protect heart tissue.

- Stable Blood Sugar Levels Maintaining stable blood sugar levels is important for preventing complications associated with AFib, particularly for individuals with diabetes or prediabetes. An AFib diet focuses on low glycemic index (GI) foods that release glucose slowly into the bloodstream, avoiding spikes and crashes in blood sugar levels.

Foods such as whole grains, legumes, and non-starchy vegetables are excellent choices for keeping blood sugar stable. Avoiding refined carbohydrates and sugary snacks helps prevent insulin resistance and supports overall metabolic health.

CHAPTER 2

BREAKFAST RECIPES

Berry Quinoa Breakfast Bowl

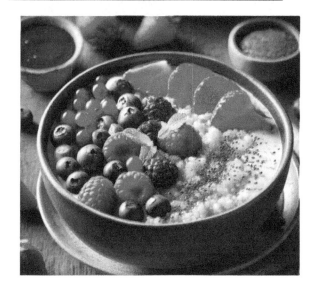

Serves: 1

Cooking Time: 20 minutes

Ingredients and Portions/Measurements:

- Quinoa: 1/3 cup (Rich in protein, fibre, and essential amino acids; a healthy carb that's AFib friendly)
- Water: 2/3 cup (For cooking quinoa)
- Fresh Mixed Berries (strawberries, blueberries, raspberries): 1/2 cup (High in antioxidants, vitamins, and low in sugar; beneficial for heart health)

- Chia Seeds: 1 tablespoon (High in omega-3 fatty acids and fiber, supports heart health)
- Cinnamon: 1/4 teaspoon (Anti-inflammatory properties and can help regulate blood sugar levels)
- Unsweetened Almond Milk: 1/4 cup (Low in calories and fat, can be substituted with any non-dairy milk for those with nut allergies)
- Pure Maple Syrup: 1 teaspoon (Natural sweetener, use sparingly)
- Fresh Mint for garnish (optional)

Instructions:

- Rinse the quinoa under cold water to remove its natural coating, saponin, which can make it taste bitter or soapy.
- In a small saucepan, bring water and quinoa to a boil. Reduce heat to low, cover, and simmer for 15 minutes or until the quinoa is tender and the water is absorbed.
- While the quinoa is cooking, wash the mixed berries and set them aside.
- Once the quinoa is done, fluff it with a fork and transfer it to a bowl.
- Stir in the cinnamon and almond milk into the quinoa until well mixed.

- Top the quinoa with fresh mixed berries, chia seeds, and a drizzle of maple syrup.

- Garnish with fresh mint if desired.

- Enjoy your Berry Quinoa Breakfast Bowl warm or cold!

Scientific Note:

Quinoa is an excellent ingredient for those on an AFib diet due to its high protein content and essential amino acids, which support overall heart health. It's also a good source of fiber, aiding in digestion and helping maintain a healthy weight.

Mixed berries are loaded with antioxidants, which protect the heart by reducing inflammation and oxidative stress. Chia seeds are a fantastic source of omega-3 fatty acids, which have been shown to help reduce inflammation and support cardiovascular health.

Cinnamon not only adds flavour but also has the potential to assist in blood sugar control, important for those managing heart health. This meal is carefully crafted to support heart health and provide a nutrient-dense start to the day.

Nutritional Information (per serving):

- Calories: ~300
- Protein: 8-10g
- Total Fat: 5-7g (mainly from chia seeds, very minimal from almond milk)
- Fiber: 5-7g
- Sodium: Low

Blueberry Chia Pudding

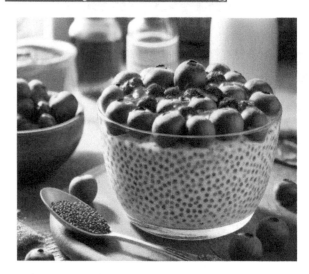

Serves: 1

Cooking Time: 5 minutes (plus overnight refrigeration)

Ingredients and Portions/Measurements:

- Chia Seeds: 3 tablespoons (High in omega-3 fatty acids and fiber, supports heart health)

- Unsweetened Almond Milk: 1 cup (Low in calories and fat, can be substituted with any non-dairy milk for those with nut allergies)

- Fresh Blueberries: 1/2 cup (High in antioxidants, vitamins, and low in sugar; beneficial for heart health)

- Pure Vanilla Extract: 1/2 teaspoon (Optional, adds flavor without added sugar)
- Pure Maple Syrup: 1 teaspoon (Natural sweetener, use sparingly, can be omitted for a lower sugar option)

Instructions:

- In a medium-sized bowl, combine chia seeds, almond milk, and vanilla extract. Stir well to ensure the seeds are evenly distributed.
- Cover the bowl and refrigerate overnight or for at least 4 hours to allow the chia seeds to absorb the liquid and form a pudding-like consistency.
- Before serving, give the chia pudding a good stir to break up any clumps.
- Top the chia pudding with fresh blueberries and drizzle with maple syrup if desired.
- Enjoy your Blueberry Chia Pudding chilled.

Scientific Note:

Chia seeds are an excellent source of omega-3 fatty acids, which have been shown to reduce inflammation and support cardiovascular health. They are also high in fiber, which aids in digestion and helps maintain a healthy weight—both important factors in managing AFib.

Blueberries are rich in antioxidants, particularly anthocyanins, which help protect the heart by reducing oxidative stress and inflammation. They are also low in sugar, making them a heart-healthy fruit choice.

Unsweetened almond milk is a low-calorie, low-fat alternative to dairy milk, suitable for those with lactose intolerance or nut allergies (if substituted with another non-dairy milk). The combination of chia seeds and almond milk provides a nutrient-dense, heart-friendly base for this breakfast.

Nutritional Information (per serving):

- Calories: ˜180
- Protein: 5g
- Total Fat: 9g (mainly from chia seeds)
- Fiber: 12g
- Sodium: Low (depending on the brand of almond milk used)
- Omega-3 Fatty Acids: ˜4g

Spinach and Tomato Egg White Omelette

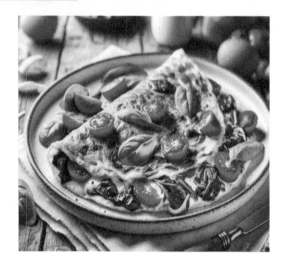

Serves: 1

Cooking Time: 10 minutes

Ingredients and Portions/Measurements:

- Egg Whites: 3 large egg whites (High in protein, low in fat, AFib friendly)
- Fresh Spinach: 1 cup (Packed with vitamins and minerals, supports heart health)
- Cherry Tomatoes (halved): 1/2 cup (Rich in antioxidants, particularly lycopene, beneficial for heart health)
- Olive Oil: 1 teaspoon (Healthy fat, contains omega-3 fatty acids, supports cardiovascular health)
- Salt: A pinch (optional, use sparingly to keep sodium intake low)
- Black Pepper: A pinch (Anti-inflammatory properties)
- Fresh Basil (optional): For garnish

Instructions:

- In a non-stick skillet, heat olive oil over medium heat.
- Add the fresh spinach to the skillet and sauté until wilted, about 2-3 minutes.
- Add the cherry tomatoes to the skillet and cook for an additional 2 minutes until they start to soften.
- In a bowl, whisk the egg whites with a pinch of salt and black pepper.
- Pour the egg whites over the spinach and tomatoes in the skillet.
- Cook until the egg whites are set, about 3-4 minutes, gently lifting the edges with a spatula to allow uncooked egg whites to flow underneath.
- Fold the omelette in half and transfer to a plate.
- Garnish with fresh basil if desired.
- Enjoy your Spinach and Tomato Egg White Omelette warm.

Scientific Note:

Egg whites are an excellent source of high-quality protein while being low in fat, making them a heart-friendly choice for those managing AFib. They help maintain muscle mass and provide essential amino acids without contributing to cholesterol levels.

Spinach is rich in vitamins A, C, and K, as well as minerals like magnesium and potassium, which are crucial for heart health. The high potassium content helps manage blood pressure, reducing the strain on the cardiovascular system.

Cherry tomatoes are loaded with antioxidants, particularly lycopene, which has been shown to reduce inflammation and protect the heart. They also provide vitamins A and C, supporting overall health and reducing oxidative stress.

Olive oil is a source of healthy monounsaturated fats and omega-3 fatty acids, which are known to reduce inflammation and support cardiovascular health. Using olive oil instead of saturated fats can help manage cholesterol levels and improve heart function.

Nutritional Information (per serving):

- Calories: ~150
- Protein: 12g
- Total Fat: 5g (mainly from olive oil)
- Fiber: 2g
- Sodium: Low (depending on the amount of salt used)

Greek Yogurt Parfait with Flaxseed and Berries

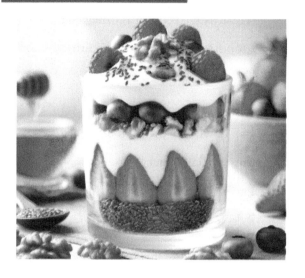

Serves: 1

Cooking Time: 5 minutes

Ingredients and Portions/Measurements:

- Plain Greek Yogurt (non-fat): 1 cup (Rich in protein, supports heart health)
- Fresh Mixed Berries (blueberries, strawberries, raspberries): 1/2 cup (High in antioxidants, vitamins, and low in sugar; beneficial for heart health)
- Flaxseed (ground): 1 tablespoon (High in omega-3 fatty acids and fiber, supports heart health)
- Honey: 1 teaspoon (Natural sweetener, use sparingly, can be omitted for a lower sugar option)

- **Vanilla Extract:** 1/2 teaspoon (Optional, adds flavor without added sugar)
- **Walnuts (chopped):** 1 tablespoon (Healthy fats, contains omega-3 fatty acids, supports cardiovascular health)

Instructions:

- In a bowl, mix the plain Greek yogurt with the vanilla extract if using.
- Layer the yogurt in a serving glass or bowl.
- Add a layer of fresh mixed berries on top of the yogurt.
- Sprinkle the ground flaxseed over the berries.
- Drizzle with honey if desired.
- Top with chopped walnuts for added crunch and healthy fats.
- Serve immediately and enjoy your Greek Yogurt Parfait with Flaxseed and Berries.

Scientific Note:

Plain Greek yogurt is an excellent source of high-quality protein and probiotics, which are beneficial for gut health. Maintaining a healthy gut can indirectly support heart health by reducing inflammation and supporting the immune system.

Mixed berries are rich in antioxidants, particularly anthocyanins, which help protect the heart by reducing oxidative stress and inflammation. They are also low in sugar, making them a heart-healthy fruit choice.

Flaxseeds are a fantastic source of omega-3 fatty acids and fiber, both of which support cardiovascular health by reducing inflammation and helping to maintain healthy cholesterol levels.

Walnuts provide healthy fats, particularly omega-3 fatty acids, which are known to reduce inflammation and support cardiovascular health. They also add a satisfying crunch to the parfait.

Nutritional Information (per serving):

- Calories: ~300
- Protein: 20g
- Total Fat: 12g (mainly from walnuts and flaxseed)
- Fiber: 7g
- Sodium: Low (depending on the brand of Greek yogurt used)

Apple Cinnamon Overnight Oats

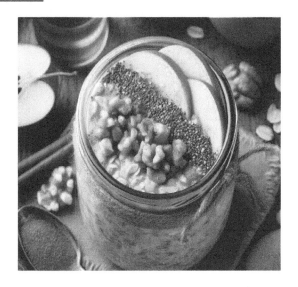

Serves: 1

Cooking Time: 10 minutes (plus overnight refrigeration)

Ingredients and Portions/Measurements:

- **Old-Fashioned Oats:** 1/2 cup (Rich in fiber, supports heart health)
- **Unsweetened Almond Milk:** 1/2 cup (Low in calories and fat, can be substituted with any non-dairy milk for those with nut allergies)
- **Apple (diced):** 1/2 medium apple (High in fiber and antioxidants, supports heart health)
- **Chia Seeds:** 1 tablespoon (High in omega-3 fatty acids and fiber, supports heart health)
- **Cinnamon:** 1/2 teaspoon (Anti-inflammatory properties, helps regulate blood sugar levels)
- **Pure Maple Syrup:** 1 teaspoon (Natural sweetener, use sparingly)
- **Vanilla Extract:** 1/4 teaspoon (Optional, adds flavor without added sugar)
- **Walnuts (chopped):** 1 tablespoon (Healthy fats, contains omega-3 fatty acids, supports cardiovascular health)

Instructions:

- In a jar or container with a lid, combine old-fashioned oats, chia seeds, and cinnamon.
- Add the unsweetened almond milk and vanilla extract (if using) to the dry ingredients and stir well to combine.
- Stir in the diced apple and pure maple syrup.
- Cover the jar or container and refrigerate overnight, or for at least 4 hours, to allow the oats to absorb the liquid and soften.
- In the morning, stir the oats to make sure everything is well mixed.
- Top with chopped walnuts for added crunch and healthy fats.

- Serve chilled and enjoy your Apple Cinnamon Overnight Oats.

Scientific Note:

Old-fashioned oats are an excellent source of dietary fiber, particularly beta-glucan, which helps manage blood cholesterol levels and supports heart health. Fiber also aids in digestion and helps maintain a healthy weight, which is important for managing AFib.

Apples are rich in dietary fiber and antioxidants, particularly flavonoids, which help reduce inflammation and protect the heart. The fiber in apples helps regulate blood sugar levels and promotes a healthy digestive system.

Chia seeds are a fantastic source of omega-3 fatty acids and fiber, both of which support cardiovascular health by reducing inflammation and helping to maintain healthy cholesterol levels. They also provide protein and essential minerals.

Cinnamon has anti-inflammatory properties and can help regulate blood sugar levels, which is important for overall health and managing heart conditions.

Walnuts provide healthy fats, particularly omega-3 fatty acids, which are known to reduce inflammation and support cardiovascular health. They also add a satisfying crunch to the oats.

Nutritional Information (per serving):

- Calories: ~300
- Protein: 8g
- Total Fat: 14g (mainly from chia seeds and walnuts)
- Fiber: 8g
- Sodium: Low (depending on the brand of almond milk used)

Smoked Salmon and Avocado Toast

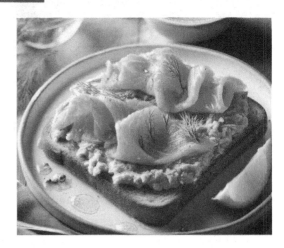

Serves: 1

Cooking Time: 10 minutes

Ingredients and Portions/Measurements:

- Whole Grain Bread: 1 slice (Rich in fiber, supports heart health)
- Avocado (mashed): 1/2 medium avocado (Healthy fat, contains omega-3 fatty acids, supports cardiovascular health)

18

- Smoked Salmon: 2 ounces (Rich in omega-3 fatty acids, supports heart health)
- Lemon Juice: 1 teaspoon (Adds flavor and vitamin C)
- Olive Oil: 1/2 teaspoon (Healthy fat, contains omega-3 fatty acids, supports cardiovascular health)
- Salt: A pinch (optional, use sparingly to keep sodium intake low)
- Black Pepper: A pinch (Anti-inflammatory properties)
- Fresh Dill (optional): For garnish

Instructions:

- Toast the whole grain bread until it is golden brown and crispy.
- In a small bowl, mash the avocado with a fork until smooth. Stir in the lemon juice to prevent browning and add a pinch of salt and black pepper for taste.
- Spread the mashed avocado evenly over the toasted bread.
- Top with smoked salmon slices.
- Drizzle with olive oil for added flavor and healthy fats.
- Garnish with fresh dill if desired.
- Serve immediately and enjoy your Smoked Salmon and Avocado Toast.

Scientific Note:

Whole grain bread is an excellent source of dietary fiber, which helps manage blood cholesterol levels and supports heart health. Fiber also aids in digestion and helps maintain a healthy weight, which is important for managing AFib.

Avocado is rich in monounsaturated fats, particularly omega-3 fatty acids, which are known to reduce inflammation and support cardiovascular health. Avocados also provide potassium, which helps regulate blood pressure—a critical factor in managing AFib.

Smoked salmon is a fantastic source of omega-3 fatty acids, which help reduce inflammation and support heart health. It's also high in protein and provides important vitamins and minerals, such as vitamin D and selenium.

Lemon juice adds a refreshing flavor and is a good source of vitamin C, which has antioxidant properties that support overall health.

Nutritional Information (per serving):

- Calories: ~350
- Protein: 15g
- Total Fat: 25g (mainly from avocado, smoked salmon, and olive oil)
- Fiber: 8g
- Sodium: Low (depending on the amount of salt used and the brand of smoked salmon)

Spinach and Mushroom Egg White Scramble

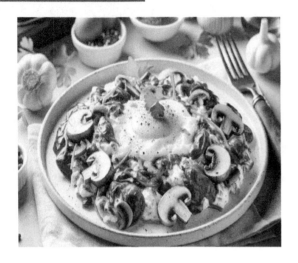

Serves: 1

Cooking Time: 10 minutes

Ingredients and Portions/Measurements:

- Egg Whites: 3 large egg whites (High in protein, low in fat, AFib friendly)
- Fresh Spinach: 1 cup (Packed with vitamins and minerals, supports heart health)
- Mushrooms (sliced): 1/2 cup (Low in calories, high in antioxidants)
- Olive Oil: 1 teaspoon (Healthy fat, contains omega-3 fatty acids, supports cardiovascular health)
- Onion (diced): 1/4 cup (Anti-inflammatory properties, supports heart health)
- Garlic (minced): 1 clove (Anti-inflammatory properties)
- Salt: A pinch (optional, use sparingly to keep sodium intake low)
- Black Pepper: A pinch (Anti-inflammatory properties)
- Fresh Parsley (optional): For garnish

Instructions:

- Heat olive oil in a non-stick skillet over medium heat.
- Add the diced onion and mushrooms to the skillet and cook for about 5 minutes until the vegetables are tender.
- Add the minced garlic and cook for 1 minute until fragrant.
- Stir in the fresh spinach and cook until wilted, about 2-3 minutes.
- In a bowl, whisk the egg whites with a pinch of salt and black pepper.
- Pour the egg whites over the vegetables in the skillet.
- Cook, stirring gently, until the egg whites are set, about 2-3 minutes.
- Serve immediately and garnish with fresh parsley if desired.
- Enjoy your Spinach and Mushroom Egg White Scramble warm.

Scientific Note:

Egg whites are an excellent source of high-quality protein while being low in fat, making them a heart-friendly choice for those managing AFib. They help maintain muscle mass and provide essential amino acids without contributing to cholesterol levels.

Spinach is rich in vitamins A, C, and K, as well as minerals like magnesium and potassium, which are crucial for heart health. The high potassium content helps manage blood pressure, reducing the strain on the cardiovascular system.

Mushrooms are low in calories but high in antioxidants, which help protect the heart by reducing oxidative stress and inflammation. They also provide important nutrients like selenium and vitamin D.

Garlic and onions have anti-inflammatory properties and are known to support heart health by improving blood circulation and reducing blood pressure.

Nutritional Information (per serving):

- Calories: ~150
- Protein: 12g
- Total Fat: 5g (mainly from olive oil)
- Fiber: 2g
- Sodium: Low (depending on the amount of salt used)

Tropical Smoothie Bowl

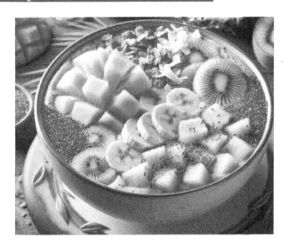

Serves: 1

Cooking Time: 10 minutes

Ingredients and Portions/Measurements:

- Frozen Pineapple Chunks: 1/2 cup (Rich in vitamin C and antioxidants, supports heart health)
- Frozen Mango Chunks: 1/2 cup (High in vitamins A and C, supports immune function and heart health)
- Banana: 1 small (High in potassium, helps regulate blood pressure)
- Unsweetened Coconut Milk: 1/2 cup (Low in calories, provides a tropical flavor)
- Chia Seeds: 1 tablespoon (High in omega-3 fatty acids and fiber, supports heart health)
- Granola (low-sugar): 2 tablespoons (Adds crunch and fiber, supports heart health)

- **Fresh Kiwi (sliced):** 1 (High in vitamin C and antioxidants)
- **Unsweetened Shredded Coconut:** 1 tablespoon (Provides healthy fats, supports cardiovascular health)

Instructions:

- In a blender, combine the frozen pineapple chunks, frozen mango chunks, banana, and unsweetened coconut milk.
- Blend until smooth and creamy. If the mixture is too thick, add a little more coconut milk until you reach your desired consistency.
- Pour the smoothie into a bowl.
- Top with chia seeds, granola, fresh kiwi slices, and unsweetened shredded coconut.
- Serve immediately and enjoy your Tropical Smoothie Bowl.

Scientific Note:

Pineapple is rich in vitamin C and antioxidants, which help reduce inflammation and support heart health. The bromelain enzyme in pineapple can aid in digestion and reduce the risk of blood clots.

Mango is high in vitamins A and C, which support immune function and heart health. It also provides fiber, which helps regulate blood sugar levels and promotes a healthy digestive system.

Bananas are an excellent source of potassium, which helps regulate blood pressure and maintain electrolyte balance, crucial for managing AFib. They also provide natural sweetness and a creamy texture to the smoothie.

Chia seeds are a fantastic source of omega-3 fatty acids and fiber, both of which support cardiovascular health by reducing inflammation and helping to maintain healthy cholesterol levels.

Coconut milk provides a tropical flavor while being low in calories and fat. It adds creaminess to the smoothie without contributing to cholesterol levels.

Kiwi is high in vitamin C and antioxidants, which help protect the heart by reducing oxidative stress and inflammation. It also provides fiber, which aids in digestion and helps maintain a healthy weight.

Granola adds crunch and fiber to the smoothie bowl, supporting heart health and providing a satisfying texture.

Nutritional Information (per serving):

- Calories: ~300
- Protein: 5g
- Total Fat: 12g (mainly from chia seeds and coconut)
- Fiber: 8g

- Sodium: Low
- Omega-3 Fatty Acids: ~2g

Apple and Almond Butter Breakfast Wrap

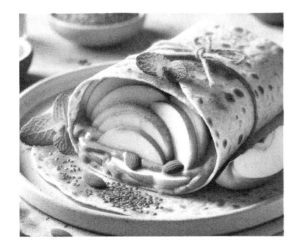

Serves: 1

Cooking Time: 5 minutes

Ingredients and Portions/Measurements:

- Whole Wheat Tortilla: 1 (Rich in fiber, supports heart health)
- Apple (thinly sliced): 1/2 medium apple (High in fiber and antioxidants, supports heart health)
- Almond Butter: 2 tablespoons (Healthy fat, contains omega-3 fatty acids, supports cardiovascular health)
- Ground Flaxseed: 1 tablespoon (High in omega-3 fatty acids and fiber, supports heart health)
- Cinnamon: 1/4 teaspoon (Anti-inflammatory properties, helps regulate blood sugar levels)
- Honey: 1 teaspoon (Natural sweetener, use sparingly)
- Fresh Mint (optional): For garnish

Instructions:

- Lay the whole wheat tortilla flat on a clean surface.
- Spread the almond butter evenly over the tortilla.
- Arrange the thinly sliced apples on top of the almond butter.
- Sprinkle with ground flaxseed and cinnamon.
- Drizzle with honey if desired.
- Roll up the tortilla tightly to form a wrap.
- Cut the wrap in half if desired.
- Garnish with fresh mint if desired.
- Serve immediately and enjoy your Apple and Almond Butter Breakfast Wrap.

Scientific Note:

Whole wheat tortillas are an excellent source of dietary fiber, which helps manage blood cholesterol levels and supports heart health. Fiber also aids in digestion and helps maintain a healthy weight, which is important for managing AFib.

Almond butter is rich in monounsaturated fats, particularly omega-3 fatty acids, which are known to reduce inflammation and support cardiovascular health. Almonds also provide protein, fiber, and essential minerals like magnesium.

Apples are high in dietary fiber and antioxidants, particularly flavonoids, which help reduce inflammation and protect the heart. The fiber in apples helps regulate blood sugar levels and promotes a healthy digestive system.

Ground flaxseed is a fantastic source of omega-3 fatty acids and fiber, both of which support cardiovascular health by reducing inflammation and helping to maintain healthy cholesterol levels.

Cinnamon has anti-inflammatory properties and can help regulate blood sugar levels, which is important for overall health and managing heart conditions.

Honey is a natural sweetener that can be used sparingly to add flavor. It has antioxidant properties but should be used in moderation to keep sugar intake low.

Nutritional Information (per serving):

- Calories: ~350
- Protein: 10g
- Total Fat: 20g (mainly from almond butter and flaxseed)
- Fiber: 8g

- Sodium: Low (depending on the amount of salt in the tortilla)

CONGRATULATION GOING TO LUNCH RECIPES

Dear Reader,

Congratulations on completing the breakfast recipes section! I hope you found joy and deliciousness in every bite. Your culinary journey has just begun, and I'm thrilled to have you continue with us.

Your feedback is invaluable, so please leave an honest review—your thoughts will help make this book even better.

Now, let's dive into the next chapter: lunch recipes. Get ready for more mouth-watering dishes that will brighten up your midday meals.

CHAPTER 3

LUNCH RECIPES

Grilled Chicken and Quinoa Salad

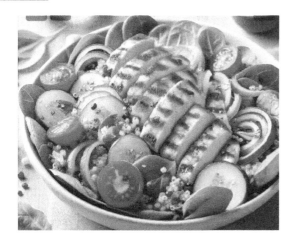

Serves: 1

Cooking Time: 30 minutes

Ingredients and Portions/Measurements:

- Boneless, Skinless Chicken Breast: 4 ounces (Lean protein, AFib friendly)
- Quinoa: 1/4 cup (Rich in protein, fiber, and essential amino acids; a healthy carb that's AFib friendly)
- Water: 1/2 cup (For cooking quinoa)
- Baby Spinach: 1 cup (Packed with vitamins and minerals, supports heart health)
- Cherry Tomatoes (halved): 1/4 cup (Rich in antioxidants, particularly lycopene, beneficial for heart health)
- Cucumber (diced): 1/4 cup (Hydrating and low in calories, supports overall health)
- Red Onion (thinly sliced): 2 tablespoons (Anti-inflammatory properties, supports heart health)
- Olive Oil: 1 tablespoon (Healthy fat, contains omega-3 fatty acids, supports cardiovascular health)
- Lemon Juice: 1 tablespoon (Adds flavor and vitamin C)
- Salt: A pinch (optional, use sparingly to keep sodium intake low)
- Black Pepper: A pinch (Anti-inflammatory properties)
- Fresh Parsley (chopped, optional): For garnish

Instructions:

- Cook the quinoa: Rinse the quinoa under cold water to remove its natural coating, saponin, which can make it taste bitter or soapy. In a small saucepan, bring water and quinoa to a boil. Reduce heat to low, cover, and simmer for 12-15 minutes or until the quinoa is tender and the water is absorbed.

- **Grill the chicken:** While the quinoa is cooking, season the chicken breast with a pinch of salt and black pepper. Grill the chicken over medium heat for about 6-7 minutes on each side, or until fully cooked and no longer pink in the center. Let it rest for a few minutes, then slice into thin strips.
- **Prepare the salad:** In a large bowl, combine the baby spinach, cherry tomatoes, cucumber, and red onion.
- Add the cooked quinoa to the salad and toss to combine.
- **Dress the salad:** In a small bowl, whisk together the olive oil and lemon juice. Pour the dressing over the salad and toss to coat.
- Top with grilled chicken slices.
- Garnish with fresh parsley if desired.
- Serve immediately and enjoy your Grilled Chicken and Quinoa Salad.

Scientific Note:

Chicken breast is a lean protein source that supports muscle maintenance and repair. It is low in fat and helps keep you feeling full, which can aid in weight management—a crucial aspect of managing AFib.

Quinoa is a complete protein, containing all nine essential amino acids. It is also rich in fiber, which helps regulate cholesterol levels and supports digestive health, making it an excellent addition to an AFib-friendly diet.

Spinach is packed with vitamins A, C, and K, as well as minerals like magnesium and potassium, which are important for heart health. The high potassium content helps manage blood pressure, reducing the strain on the cardiovascular system.

Cherry tomatoes are loaded with antioxidants, particularly lycopene, which has been shown to reduce inflammation and protect the heart. They also provide vitamins A and C, supporting overall health and reducing oxidative stress.

Nutritional Information (per serving):

- Calories: ~350
- Protein: 30g
- Total Fat: 15g (mainly from olive oil and chicken)
- Fiber: 5g
- Sodium: Low (depending on the amount of salt used)

Lentil and Vegetable Soup

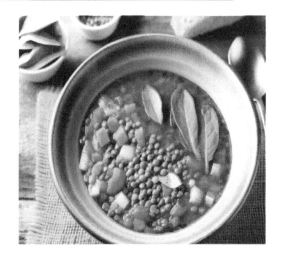

Serves: 1

Cooking Time: 40 minutes

Ingredients and Portions/Measurements:

- Green or Brown Lentils: 1/4 cup (Rich in protein and fiber, supports heart health)
- Water or Low-Sodium Vegetable Broth: 2 cups (For cooking lentils and vegetables)
- Olive Oil: 1 teaspoon (Healthy fat, contains omega-3 fatty acids, supports cardiovascular health)
- Onion (diced): 1/4 cup (Anti-inflammatory properties, supports heart health)
- Carrot (diced): 1/2 medium carrot (High in antioxidants, supports immune function and heart health)
- Celery (diced): 1 stalk (Rich in vitamins and minerals, supports heart health)

- Garlic (minced): 1 clove (Anti-inflammatory properties)
- Zucchini (diced): 1/2 small zucchini (Low in calories, supports overall health)
- Tomato (diced): 1 small tomato (Rich in antioxidants, particularly lycopene, supports heart health)
- Spinach: 1 cup (Packed with vitamins and minerals, supports heart health)
- Bay Leaf: 1 (For flavor)
- Dried Thyme: 1/2 teaspoon (Anti-inflammatory properties)
- Salt: A pinch (optional, use sparingly to keep sodium intake low)
- Black Pepper: A pinch (Anti-inflammatory properties)
- Fresh Parsley (optional): For garnish

Instructions:

- Rinse the lentils under cold water and set aside.
- In a large pot, heat olive oil over medium heat.
- Add the diced onion, carrot, and celery to the pot and sauté for about 5 minutes, until the vegetables start to soften.
- Add the minced garlic and cook for another 1 minute until fragrant.

- Stir in the diced zucchini, tomato, and lentils. Add the water or low-sodium vegetable broth, bay leaf, and dried thyme.

- Bring the mixture to a boil, then reduce heat to low and simmer for 25-30 minutes, until the lentils are tender.

- Add the spinach and cook for another 5 minutes until wilted.

- Season with a pinch of salt and black pepper to taste.

- Remove the bay leaf before serving.

- Garnish with fresh parsley if desired.

- Serve warm and enjoy your Lentil and Vegetable Soup.

Scientific Note:

Lentils are an excellent source of plant-based protein and dietary fiber, which help manage blood cholesterol levels and support heart health. Fiber also aids in digestion and helps maintain a healthy weight, which is important for managing AFib.

Garlic has anti-inflammatory properties and is known to support heart health by improving blood circulation and reducing blood pressure.

Zucchini is low in calories but high in essential nutrients, including vitamins A and C, which support overall health and reduce oxidative stress.

Spinach is packed with vitamins A, C, and K, as well as minerals like magnesium and potassium, which are important for heart health. The high potassium content helps manage blood pressure, reducing the strain on the cardiovascular system.

Nutritional Information (per serving):

- Calories: ~250

- Protein: 12g

- Total Fat: 5g (mainly from olive oil)

- Fiber: 12g

- Sodium: Low (depending on the amount of salt used)

Chickpea and Spinach Stew

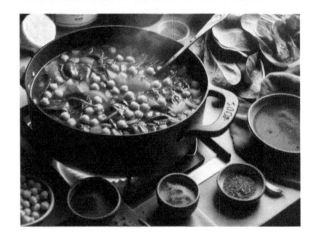

Serves: 1

Cooking Time: 25 minutes

Ingredients and Portions/Measurements:

- Olive Oil: 1 teaspoon (Healthy fat, contains omega-3 fatty acids, supports cardiovascular health)
- Onion (diced): 1/4 cup (Anti-inflammatory properties, supports heart health)
- Garlic (minced): 1 clove (Anti-inflammatory properties)
- Tomato (diced): 1 small (Rich in antioxidants, particularly lycopene, supports heart health)
- Canned Chickpeas (drained and rinsed): 1/2 cup (Rich in protein and fiber, supports heart health)
- Spinach: 1 cup (Packed with vitamins and minerals, supports heart health)
- Vegetable Broth (low-sodium): 1 cup (For cooking chickpeas and vegetables)
- Cumin: 1/2 teaspoon (Anti-inflammatory properties)
- Turmeric: 1/4 teaspoon (Anti-inflammatory and antioxidant properties)
- Salt: A pinch (optional, use sparingly to keep sodium intake low)
- Black Pepper: A pinch (Anti-inflammatory properties)
- Lemon Juice: 1 teaspoon (Adds flavor and vitamin C)
- Fresh Cilantro (optional): For garnish

Instructions:

- In a medium-sized pot, heat olive oil over medium heat.
- Add the diced onion and sauté for about 5 minutes until it becomes translucent.
- Add the minced garlic and cook for another 1 minute until fragrant.
- Stir in the diced tomato and cook for 2-3 minutes until it starts to break down.
- Add the canned chickpeas, vegetable broth, cumin, and turmeric. Bring the mixture to a simmer and cook for 10 minutes.
- Stir in the spinach and cook for another 5 minutes until wilted.
- Season with a pinch of salt and black pepper to taste.
- Stir in the lemon juice for added flavor.
- Garnish with fresh cilantro if desired.
- Serve warm and enjoy your Chickpea and Spinach Stew.

Scientific Note:

Chickpeas are an excellent source of plant-based protein and dietary fiber, which help manage blood cholesterol levels and support heart health. Fiber also aids in digestion and helps maintain a healthy weight, which is important for managing AFib.

Spinach is packed with vitamins A, C, and K, as well as minerals like magnesium and potassium, which are important for heart health. The high potassium content helps manage blood pressure, reducing the strain on the cardiovascular system.

Tomatoes are rich in antioxidants, particularly lycopene, which has been shown to reduce inflammation and protect the heart. They also provide vitamins A and C, supporting overall health and reducing oxidative stress.

Nutritional Information (per serving):

- Calories: ~300
- Protein: 12g
- Total Fat: 7g (mainly from olive oil)
- Fiber: 10g
- Sodium: Low (depending on the amount of salt used)

Mediterranean Stuffed Bell Peppers

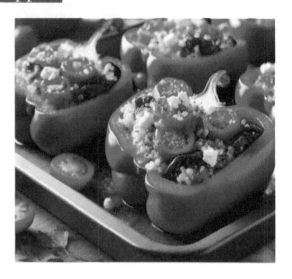

Serves: 1

Cooking Time: 35 minutes

Ingredients and Portions/Measurements:

- Red Bell Pepper (halved and seeded): 1 large (Rich in vitamins A and C, supports heart health)
- Quinoa: 1/4 cup (Rich in protein, fiber, and essential amino acids; a healthy carb that's AFib friendly)
- Water: 1/2 cup (For cooking quinoa)
- Olive Oil: 1 teaspoon (Healthy fat, contains omega-3 fatty acids, supports cardiovascular health)
- Onion (diced): 1/4 cup (Anti-inflammatory properties, supports heart health)

- Garlic (minced): 1 clove (Anti-inflammatory properties)
- Cherry Tomatoes (halved): 1/4 cup (Rich in antioxidants, particularly lycopene, supports heart health)
- Spinach: 1 cup (Packed with vitamins and minerals, supports heart health)
- Feta Cheese (crumbled): 2 tablespoons (Rich in calcium and protein, can be omitted or substituted with a dairy-free alternative if needed)
- Dried Oregano: 1/2 teaspoon (Anti-inflammatory properties)
- Salt: A pinch (optional, use sparingly to keep sodium intake low)
- Black Pepper: A pinch (Anti-inflammatory properties)
- Fresh Parsley (optional): For garnish

Instructions:

- Preheat the oven to 375°F (190°C).
- Cook the quinoa: Rinse the quinoa under cold water to remove its natural coating, saponin, which can make it taste bitter or soapy. In a small saucepan, bring water and quinoa to a boil. Reduce heat to low, cover, and simmer for 12-15 minutes or until the quinoa is tender and the water is absorbed.
- Prepare the bell pepper: While the quinoa is cooking, place the bell pepper halves cut-side up on a baking sheet.
- In a medium-sized skillet, heat olive oil over medium heat.
- Add the diced onion and sauté for about 5 minutes until it becomes translucent.
- Add the minced garlic and cook for another 1 minute until fragrant.
- Stir in the cherry tomatoes and spinach and cook for 2-3 minutes until the spinach is wilted.
- Mix the cooked quinoa into the skillet with the vegetables. Add the dried oregano, salt, and black pepper.
- Spoon the quinoa mixture into the bell pepper halves.
- Top with crumbled feta cheese.
- Bake in the preheated oven for 15-20 minutes, until the bell peppers are tender and the cheese is slightly browned.
- Garnish with fresh parsley if desired.
- Serve warm and enjoy your Mediterranean Stuffed Bell Peppers.

Scientific Note:

Quinoa is an excellent source of high-quality protein and essential amino acids, making it a heart-friendly choice for those managing AFib. It is also rich in dietary fiber, which helps regulate cholesterol levels and supports digestive health.

Red bell peppers are high in vitamins A and C, which have antioxidant properties that help protect the heart by reducing oxidative stress and inflammation. They also add a sweet and satisfying flavor to the dish.

Spinach is packed with vitamins A, C, and K, as well as minerals like magnesium and potassium, which are important for heart health. The high potassium content helps manage blood pressure, reducing the strain on the cardiovascular system.

Cherry tomatoes are rich in antioxidants, particularly lycopene, which has been shown to reduce inflammation and protect the heart. They also provide vitamins A and C, supporting overall health and reducing oxidative stress.

Feta cheese adds a creamy texture and flavor to the dish while providing calcium and protein. However, it should be used sparingly due to its sodium content.

Nutritional Information (per serving):

- Calories: ~300
- Protein: 12g
- Total Fat: 12g (mainly from olive oil and feta cheese)
- Fiber: 6g

- Sodium: Low to moderate (depending on the amount of salt used and the feta cheese)

Grilled Salmon with Mango Avocado Salsa

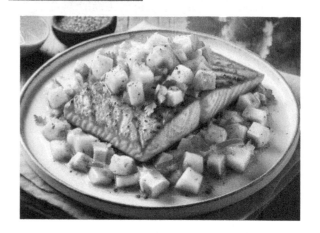

Serves: 1

Cooking Time: 20 minutes

Ingredients and Portions/Measurements:

- Salmon Fillet: 4 ounces (Rich in omega-3 fatty acids, supports cardiovascular health)
- Olive Oil: 1 teaspoon (Healthy fat, supports heart health)
- Salt: A pinch (optional, use sparingly to keep sodium intake low)
- Black Pepper: A pinch (Anti-inflammatory properties)
- Garlic Powder: 1/4 teaspoon (Anti-inflammatory properties)

- Lime Juice: 1 tablespoon (Adds flavor and vitamin C)

Mango Avocado Salsa:

- Mango (diced): 1/4 cup (Rich in vitamins A and C, supports immune function and heart health)
- Avocado (diced): 1/2 medium avocado (Healthy fat, contains omega-3 fatty acids, supports cardiovascular health)
- Red Onion (diced): 1 tablespoon (Anti-inflammatory properties)
- Cilantro (chopped): 1 tablespoon (Adds flavor and antioxidants)
- Lime Juice: 1 tablespoon (Adds flavor and vitamin C)

Instructions:

- Preheat the grill to medium-high heat.
- Season the salmon fillet with olive oil, salt, black pepper, and garlic powder.
- Grill the salmon for about 4-5 minutes on each side, or until it flakes easily with a fork.
- While the salmon is grilling, prepare the mango avocado salsa: In a medium bowl, combine diced mango, diced avocado, red onion, cilantro, and lime juice. Mix gently to combine.
- Remove the salmon from the grill and squeeze lime juice over the top.
- Serve the grilled salmon topped with the mango avocado salsa.
- Enjoy your Grilled Salmon with Mango Avocado Salsa warm.

Scientific Note:

Salmon is an excellent source of high-quality protein and omega-3 fatty acids, which are known to reduce inflammation and support cardiovascular health. Omega-3 fatty acids help lower blood pressure, reduce triglycerides, and prevent the formation of blood clots.

Mango is rich in vitamins A and C, which support immune function and heart health. It also provides dietary fiber, which helps regulate blood sugar levels and promotes a healthy digestive system.

Avocado is rich in monounsaturated fats, particularly omega-3 fatty acids, which help reduce inflammation and support cardiovascular health. Avocados also provide potassium, which helps regulate blood pressure—a critical factor in managing AFib.

Red onions have anti-inflammatory properties and are known to support heart health by improving blood circulation and reducing blood pressure.

Olive oil is a source of healthy monounsaturated fats and omega-3 fatty acids, which help reduce inflammation and support cardiovascular health. Using olive oil instead of saturated fats can help manage cholesterol levels and improve heart function.

Lime juice adds a refreshing flavor and is a good source of vitamin C, which has antioxidant properties that support overall health.

Nutritional Information (per serving):

- Calories: ~350
- Protein: 25g
- Total Fat: 20g (mainly from salmon, avocado, and olive oil)
- Fiber: 5g
- Sodium: Low (depending on the amount of salt used)

Zucchini Noodles with Pesto and Cherry Tomatoes

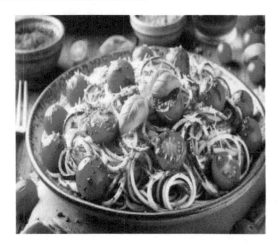

Serves: 1

Cooking Time: 20 minutes

Ingredients and Portions/Measurements:

- Zucchini: 1 large (Spiralized into noodles, low in calories and high in fiber, supports heart health)
- Olive Oil: 1 teaspoon (Healthy fat, supports cardiovascular health)
- Cherry Tomatoes (halved): 1/2 cup (Rich in antioxidants, particularly lycopene, supports heart health)
- Basil Pesto: 2 tablespoons (Can be homemade or store-bought, choose a low-sodium option)
- Garlic (minced): 1 clove (Anti-inflammatory properties)
- Parmesan Cheese (grated): 1 tablespoon (Optional, for garnish)
- Salt: A pinch (optional, use sparingly to keep sodium intake low)
- Black Pepper: A pinch (Anti-inflammatory properties)
- Fresh Basil (optional): For garnish

Instructions:

- Spiralize the zucchini into noodles using a spiralizer or a vegetable peeler.
- In a large skillet, heat olive oil over medium heat.
- Add the minced garlic and sauté for about 1 minute until fragrant.

- Add the cherry tomatoes to the skillet and cook for 3-4 minutes until they start to soften.
- Add the zucchini noodles to the skillet and cook for 2-3 minutes, tossing gently until they are tender but still slightly firm.
- Stir in the basil pesto and toss to coat the zucchini noodles evenly.
- Season with a pinch of salt and black pepper to taste.
- Transfer the zucchini noodles to a serving plate.
- Garnish with grated Parmesan cheese and fresh basil if desired.
- Serve immediately and enjoy your Zucchini Noodles with Pesto and Cherry Tomatoes.

Scientific Note:

Zucchini is low in calories but high in essential nutrients, including vitamins A and C, which support overall health and reduce oxidative stress. It is also a good source of dietary fiber, which helps regulate cholesterol levels and supports digestive health.

Cherry tomatoes are rich in antioxidants, particularly lycopene, which has been shown to reduce inflammation and protect the heart. They also provide vitamins A and C, supporting overall health and reducing oxidative stress.

Basil pesto, made primarily from basil, garlic, olive oil, and nuts, provides a flavorful and heart-healthy sauce. Basil contains antioxidants and anti-inflammatory compounds that support heart health. Olive oil and nuts add healthy fats, particularly omega-3 fatty acids, which help reduce inflammation and support cardiovascular health.

Parmesan cheese adds a touch of flavor and creaminess to the dish but should be used sparingly due to its sodium content. It can be omitted or substituted with a low-sodium alternative if needed.

Nutritional Information (per serving):

- Calories: ~250
- Protein: 5g
- Total Fat: 18g (mainly from olive oil and pesto)
- Fiber: 5g
- Sodium: Low to moderate (depending on the amount of salt and Parmesan cheese used)

Sweet Potato and Black Bean Tacos

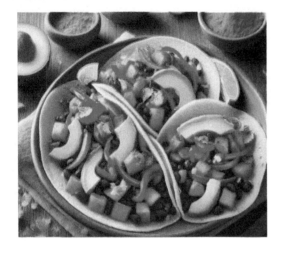

Serves: 1

Cooking Time: 30 minutes

Ingredients and Portions/Measurements:

- Olive Oil: 1 teaspoon (Healthy fat, supports cardiovascular health)
- Sweet Potato (peeled and diced): 1 small (Rich in potassium, helps regulate blood pressure)
- Black Beans (canned, drained, and rinsed): 1/2 cup (Rich in protein and fiber, supports heart health)
- Red Bell Pepper (diced): 1/4 cup (Rich in vitamins A and C, supports heart health)
- Onion (diced): 1/4 cup (Anti-inflammatory properties, supports heart health)
- Garlic (minced): 1 clove (Anti-inflammatory properties)
- Ground Cumin: 1/2 teaspoon (Anti-inflammatory properties)
- Chili Powder: 1/4 teaspoon (Anti-inflammatory properties)
- Salt: A pinch (optional, use sparingly to keep sodium intake low)
- Black Pepper: A pinch (Anti-inflammatory properties)
- Corn Tortillas: 2 small (Whole grain, supports heart health)
- Avocado (sliced): 1/4 medium avocado (Healthy fat, contains omega-3 fatty acids, supports cardiovascular health)
- Fresh Cilantro (chopped): 1 tablespoon (Adds flavor and antioxidants)
- Lime Wedges: For serving

Instructions:

- In a medium-sized skillet, heat olive oil over medium heat.
- Add the diced sweet potato to the skillet and cook for about 10 minutes, stirring occasionally, until it starts to soften.
- Add the diced red bell pepper, onion, and minced garlic to the skillet and cook for another 5 minutes until the vegetables are tender.

- Stir in the black beans, ground cumin, chili powder, salt, and black pepper. Cook for another 5 minutes until everything is well combined and heated through.
- While the filling is cooking, warm the corn tortillas in a dry skillet or microwave until pliable.
- Assemble the tacos: Divide the sweet potato and black bean mixture between the tortillas.
- Top with sliced avocado and chopped fresh cilantro.
- Serve with lime wedges on the side.
- Enjoy your Sweet Potato and Black Bean Tacos warm.

Scientific Note:

Sweet potatoes are rich in potassium, which helps regulate blood pressure and maintain electrolyte balance, crucial for managing AFib. They also provide dietary fiber and antioxidants, which support overall heart health.

Black beans are an excellent source of plant-based protein and dietary fiber, which help manage blood cholesterol levels and support heart health. Fiber also aids in digestion and helps maintain a healthy weight.

Red bell peppers are high in vitamins A and C, which have antioxidant properties that help protect the heart by reducing oxidative stress and inflammation. They also add a sweet and satisfying flavor to the dish.

Avocado is rich in monounsaturated fats, particularly omega-3 fatty acids, which help reduce inflammation and support cardiovascular health. Avocados also provide potassium, which helps regulate blood pressure.

Corn tortillas made from whole grain provide dietary fiber and essential nutrients while being low in fat. They are a heart-healthy alternative to refined grain tortillas.

Olive oil is a source of healthy monounsaturated fats and omega-3 fatty acids, which help reduce inflammation and support cardiovascular health. Using olive oil instead of saturated fats can help manage cholesterol levels and improve heart function.

Nutritional Information (per serving):

- Calories: ~350
- Protein: 10g
- Total Fat: 12g (mainly from avocado and olive oil)
- Fiber: 12g
- Sodium: Low (depending on the amount of salt used)

Chickpea and Spinach Stuffed Portobello Mushrooms

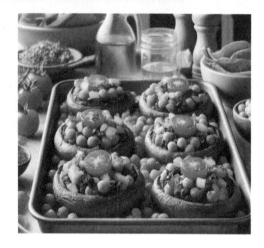

Serves: 1

Cooking Time: 25 minutes

Ingredients and Portions/Measurements:

- Large Portobello Mushrooms (stems removed): 2 (Low in calories, supports heart health)
- Olive Oil: 1 teaspoon (Healthy fat, supports cardiovascular health)
- Onion (diced): 1/4 cup (Anti-inflammatory properties, supports heart health)
- Garlic (minced): 1 clove (Anti-inflammatory properties)
- Canned Chickpeas (drained and rinsed): 1/2 cup (Rich in protein and fiber, supports heart health)
- Baby Spinach: 1 cup (Packed with vitamins and minerals, supports heart health)
- Cherry Tomatoes (halved): 1/4 cup (Rich in antioxidants, particularly lycopene, supports heart health)
- Balsamic Vinegar: 1 teaspoon (Adds flavor and antioxidants)
- Salt: A pinch (optional, use sparingly to keep sodium intake low)
- Black Pepper: A pinch (Anti-inflammatory properties)
- Fresh Parsley (chopped, optional): For garnish

Instructions:

- Preheat the oven to 375°F (190°C).
- Brush the portobello mushrooms with a little olive oil and place them on a baking sheet, gill-side up. Bake for 10 minutes until tender.
- While the mushrooms are baking, heat the remaining olive oil in a medium-sized skillet over medium heat.
- Add the diced onion and sauté for about 5 minutes until it becomes translucent.
- Add the minced garlic and cook for another 1 minute until fragrant.
- Stir in the chickpeas and cook for 3-4 minutes until heated through.

- Add the baby spinach and cook for 2-3 minutes until wilted.
- Add the cherry tomatoes and balsamic vinegar, and cook for another 2 minutes.
- Season with a pinch of salt and black pepper to taste.
- Remove the mushrooms from the oven and spoon the chickpea and spinach mixture into the mushroom caps.
- Return to the oven and bake for another 5 minutes.
- Garnish with fresh parsley if desired.
- Serve warm and enjoy your Chickpea and Spinach Stuffed Portobello Mushrooms.

Scientific Note:

Portobello mushrooms are low in calories but high in essential nutrients, including vitamins and minerals that support overall health. They also provide dietary fiber, which helps regulate cholesterol levels and supports digestive health.

Chickpeas are an excellent source of plant-based protein and dietary fiber, which help manage blood cholesterol levels and support heart health. Fiber also aids in digestion and helps maintain a healthy weight, which is important for managing AFib.

Spinach is packed with vitamins A, C, and K, as well as minerals like magnesium and potassium, which are important for heart health. The high potassium content helps manage blood pressure, reducing the strain on the cardiovascular system.

Cherry tomatoes are rich in antioxidants, particularly lycopene, which has been shown to reduce inflammation and protect the heart. They also provide vitamins A and C, supporting overall health and reducing oxidative stress.

Olive oil is a source of healthy monounsaturated fats and omega-3 fatty acids, which help reduce inflammation and support cardiovascular health. Using olive oil instead of saturated fats can help manage cholesterol levels and improve heart function.

Balsamic vinegar adds a tangy flavor and is a good source of antioxidants, which help reduce inflammation and support heart health.

Nutritional Information (per serving):

- Calories: ~250
- Protein: 10g
- Total Fat: 8g (mainly from olive oil)
- Fiber: 8g
- Sodium: Low (depending on the amount of salt used)

Lemon Herb Quinoa Salad with Grilled Shrimp

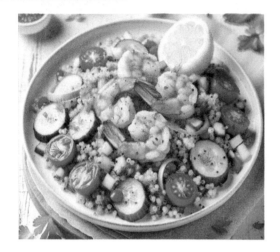

Serves: 1

Cooking Time: 30 minutes

Ingredients and Portions/Measurements:

- Quinoa: 1/4 cup (Rich in protein, fibre, and essential amino acids; a healthy carb that's AFib friendly)
- Water: 1/2 cup (For cooking quinoa)
- Olive Oil: 1 teaspoon (Healthy fat, supports cardiovascular health)
- Shrimp (peeled and deveined): 4 ounces (Rich in protein, low in fat, supports heart health)
- Garlic Powder: 1/4 teaspoon (Anti-inflammatory properties)
- Lemon Juice: 2 tablespoons (Adds flavor and vitamin C)
- Cucumber (diced): 1/4 cup (Hydrating and low in calories, supports overall health)
- Cherry Tomatoes (halved): 1/4 cup (Rich in antioxidants, particularly lycopene, supports heart health)
- Red Onion (diced): 1 tablespoon (Anti-inflammatory properties)
- Fresh Parsley (chopped): 1 tablespoon (Adds flavor and antioxidants)
- Fresh Dill (chopped): 1 tablespoon (Anti-inflammatory properties)
- Salt: A pinch (optional, use sparingly to keep sodium intake low)
- Black Pepper: A pinch (Anti-inflammatory properties)

Instructions:

- Cook the quinoa: Rinse the quinoa under cold water to remove its natural coating, saponin, which can make it taste bitter or soapy. In a small saucepan, bring water and quinoa to a boil. Reduce heat to low, cover, and simmer for 12-15 minutes or until the quinoa is tender and the water is absorbed. Let it cool.
- Prepare the shrimp: While the quinoa is cooking, heat 1/2 teaspoon of olive oil in a skillet over medium heat. Season the shrimp with garlic powder, salt, and black

pepper. Cook the shrimp for about 2-3 minutes on each side until pink and opaque. Remove from heat and set aside.

- Prepare the salad: In a large bowl, combine the cooked quinoa, diced cucumber, cherry tomatoes, red onion, fresh parsley, and fresh dill.

- Make the dressing: In a small bowl, whisk together the remaining olive oil and lemon juice.

- Assemble the salad: Pour the dressing over the quinoa mixture and toss to coat evenly.

- Add the cooked shrimp on top of the salad.

- Season with a pinch of salt and black pepper to taste.

- Serve immediately and enjoy your Lemon Herb Quinoa Salad with Grilled Shrimp.

Scientific Note:

Quinoa is an excellent source of high-quality protein and essential amino acids, making it a heart-friendly choice for those managing AFib. It is also rich in dietary fiber, which helps regulate cholesterol levels and supports digestive health.

Shrimp is a lean source of protein and provides essential nutrients like selenium and vitamin B12. It is low in fat and supports muscle maintenance and repair, which is important for overall health.

Cucumber is hydrating and low in calories while providing essential nutrients like vitamin K. It adds a refreshing crunch to the salad.

Cherry tomatoes are rich in antioxidants, particularly lycopene, which has been shown to reduce inflammation and protect the heart. They also provide vitamins A and C, supporting overall health and reducing oxidative stress.

Red onions have anti-inflammatory properties and are known to support heart health by improving blood circulation and reducing blood pressure.

Olive oil is a source of healthy monounsaturated fats and omega-3 fatty acids, which help reduce inflammation and support cardiovascular health. Using olive oil instead of saturated fats can help manage cholesterol levels and improve heart function.

Lemon juice adds a refreshing flavour and is a good source of vitamin C, which has antioxidant properties that support overall health.

Nutritional Information (per serving):

- Calories: ~350
- Protein: 20g
- Total Fat: 12g (mainly from olive oil and shrimp)
- Fiber: 5g
- Sodium: Low to moderate (depending on the amount of salt used)

CONGRATULATIONS GOING TO SNACKS AND APPETIZER RECIPES

Dear Reader,

Congratulations on completing the lunch recipes section! I hope you found joy and deliciousness in every bite. Your culinary journey has just begun, and I'm thrilled to have you continue with us.

Your feedback is invaluable, so please leave an honest review—your thoughts will help improve this book.

Now, let's dive into the next chapter: snacks and appetizer recipes. Get ready for more mouth-watering dishes that will brighten up your midday meals.

CHAPTER 4

SNACKS AND APPETIZER

Avocado and Edamame Dip with Veggie Sticks

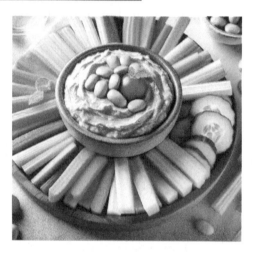

Serves: 1

Cooking Time: 15 minutes

Ingredients and Portions/Measurements:

- Edamame (shelled, cooked): 1/2 cup (Rich in protein and fiber, supports heart health)
- Avocado (mashed): 1/2 medium avocado (Healthy fat, contains omega-3 fatty acids, supports cardiovascular health)

- Garlic (minced): 1 clove (Anti-inflammatory properties)
- Lemon Juice: 1 tablespoon (Adds flavor and vitamin C)
- Olive Oil: 1 teaspoon (Healthy fat, supports cardiovascular health)
- Salt: A pinch (optional, use sparingly to keep sodium intake low)
- Black Pepper: A pinch (Anti-inflammatory properties)
- Carrot Sticks: 1/2 cup (Rich in beta-carotene and fiber, supports overall health)
- Celery Sticks: 1/2 cup (Low in calories, hydrating, supports digestive health)
- Cucumber Sticks: 1/2 cup (Hydrating, low in calories, supports overall health)

Instructions:

- In a food processor, combine the cooked edamame, mashed avocado, minced garlic, lemon juice, olive oil, salt, and black pepper.
- Blend until smooth and creamy. If the mixture is too thick, add a little water to reach the desired consistency.
- Transfer the dip to a serving bowl.
- Serve with carrot sticks, celery sticks, and cucumber sticks.

- Enjoy your Avocado and Edamame Dip with fresh veggie sticks as a heart-healthy snack.

Scientific Note:

Edamame is an excellent source of plant-based protein and dietary fiber, which help manage blood cholesterol levels and support heart health. Fiber also aids in digestion and helps maintain a healthy weight, which is important for managing AFib.

Avocado is rich in monounsaturated fats, particularly omega-3 fatty acids, which help reduce inflammation and support cardiovascular health. Avocados also provide potassium, which helps regulate blood pressure—a critical factor in managing AFib.

Garlic has anti-inflammatory properties and is known to support heart health by improving blood circulation and reducing blood pressure.

Cucumbers are hydrating and low in calories while providing essential nutrients like vitamin K. They add a refreshing crunch to the snack.

Nutritional Information (per serving):

- Calories: ~200
- Protein: 7g
- Total Fat: 15g (mainly from avocado and olive oil)
- Fiber: 8g

- Sodium: Low (depending on the amount of salt used)

Cucumber and Hummus Bites

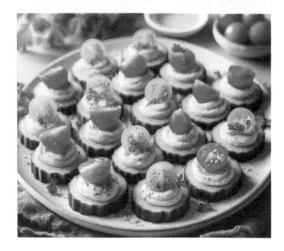

Serves: 1

Cooking Time: 10 minutes

Ingredients and Portions/Measurements:

- Cucumber: 1 large (Hydrating and low in calories, supports overall health)
- Hummus: 1/4 cup (Rich in protein and fiber, supports heart health)
- Cherry Tomatoes (halved): 4 (Rich in antioxidants, particularly lycopene, supports heart health)
- Olive Oil: 1 teaspoon (Healthy fat, supports cardiovascular health)
- Fresh Parsley (chopped): 1 tablespoon (Adds flavor and antioxidants)
- Salt: A pinch (optional, use sparingly to keep sodium intake low)

- Black Pepper: A pinch (Anti-inflammatory properties)

Instructions:

- Slice the cucumber into thick rounds.
- Spread a small amount of hummus on each cucumber slice.
- Top each slice with a halved cherry tomato.
- Drizzle with olive oil and sprinkle with salt and black pepper.
- Garnish with chopped fresh parsley.
- Serve immediately and enjoy your Cucumber and Hummus Bites as a heart-healthy snack.

Scientific Note:

Cucumbers are hydrating and low in calories while providing essential nutrients like vitamin K. They add a refreshing crunch to the snack and are excellent for maintaining hydration, which is important for heart health.

Hummus, made primarily from chickpeas, is an excellent source of plant-based protein and dietary fiber. These nutrients help manage blood cholesterol levels and support heart health. Fiber also aids in digestion and helps maintain a healthy weight, which is crucial for managing AFib.

Cherry tomatoes are rich in antioxidants, particularly lycopene, which has been shown to reduce inflammation and protect the heart. They also provide vitamins A and C, supporting overall health and reducing oxidative stress.

Olive oil is a source of healthy monounsaturated fats and omega-3 fatty acids, which help reduce inflammation and support cardiovascular health. Using olive oil instead of saturated fats can help manage cholesterol levels and improve heart function.

Parsley adds flavor and provides antioxidants that support heart health. It is also rich in vitamins A, C, and K.

Nutritional Information (per serving):

- Calories: ~150
- Protein: 4g
- Total Fat: 10g (mainly from hummus and olive oil)
- Fiber: 3g
- Sodium: Low (depending on the amount of salt used)

Roasted Red Pepper and Chickpea Mini Wraps

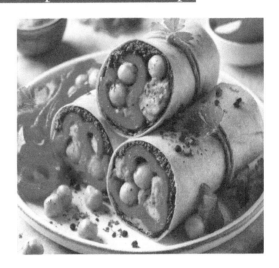

Serves: 1

Cooking Time: 15 minutes

Ingredients and Portions/Measurements:

- Whole Wheat Tortilla: 1 small (Rich in fiber, supports heart health)
- Roasted Red Pepper (sliced): 1/2 cup (Rich in vitamins A and C, supports heart health)
- Canned Chickpeas (drained and rinsed): 1/4 cup (Rich in protein and fiber, supports heart health)
- Tahini: 1 tablespoon (Healthy fat, contains omega-3 fatty acids, supports cardiovascular health)
- Lemon Juice: 1 teaspoon (Adds flavor and vitamin C)

- Garlic (minced): 1 clove (Anti-inflammatory properties)
- Olive Oil: 1 teaspoon (Healthy fat, supports cardiovascular health)
- Salt: A pinch (optional, use sparingly to keep sodium intake low)
- Black Pepper: A pinch (Anti-inflammatory properties)
- Fresh Parsley (chopped): 1 tablespoon (Adds flavor and antioxidants)

Instructions:

- In a small bowl, mash the chickpeas with a fork until slightly chunky.
- Add the tahini, lemon juice, minced garlic, olive oil, salt, and black pepper to the mashed chickpeas and mix well.
- Lay the whole wheat tortilla flat on a clean surface.
- Spread the chickpea mixture evenly over the tortilla.
- Top with sliced roasted red pepper and sprinkle with fresh parsley.
- Roll up the tortilla tightly and cut into small bite-sized pieces.
- Serve immediately and enjoy your Roasted Red Pepper and Chickpea Mini Wraps as a heart-healthy snack.

Scientific Note:

Whole wheat tortillas are an excellent source of dietary fiber, which helps manage blood cholesterol levels and supports heart health. Fiber also aids in digestion and helps maintain a healthy weight, which is important for managing AFib.

Roasted red peppers are high in vitamins A and C, which have antioxidant properties that help protect the heart by reducing oxidative stress and inflammation. They also add a sweet and satisfying flavor to the dish.

Chickpeas are an excellent source of plant-based protein and dietary fiber, which help manage blood cholesterol levels and support heart health. Fiber also aids in digestion and helps maintain a healthy weight.

Tahini, made from sesame seeds, is rich in healthy fats, particularly omega-3 fatty acids, which help reduce inflammation and support cardiovascular health. It also provides protein and essential minerals.

Nutritional Information (per serving):

- Calories: ~200
- Protein: 6g
- Total Fat: 10g (mainly from tahini and olive oil)
- Fiber: 6g
- Sodium: Low (depending on the amount of salt used)

Greek Yogurt and Herb Dip with Bell Pepper Strips

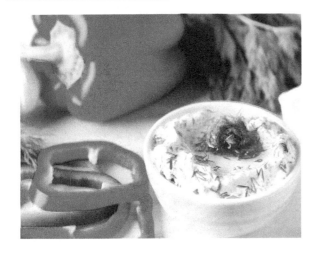

Serves: 1

Cooking Time: 10 minutes

Ingredients and Portions/Measurements:

- Plain Greek Yogurt (non-fat): 1/2 cup (Rich in protein, supports heart health)
- Fresh Dill (chopped): 1 tablespoon (Adds flavor and antioxidants)
- Fresh Parsley (chopped): 1 tablespoon (Adds flavor and antioxidants)
- Garlic (minced): 1 clove (Anti-inflammatory properties)
- Lemon Juice: 1 teaspoon (Adds flavor and vitamin C)
- Olive Oil: 1 teaspoon (Healthy fat, supports cardiovascular health)
- Salt: A pinch (optional, use sparingly to keep sodium intake low)
- Black Pepper: A pinch (Anti-inflammatory properties)
- Red Bell Pepper (sliced): 1 large (Rich in vitamins A and C, supports heart health)

Instructions:

- In a small bowl, combine the plain Greek yogurt, chopped dill, chopped parsley, minced garlic, lemon juice, olive oil, salt, and black pepper. Mix well until all ingredients are thoroughly combined.
- Transfer the yogurt dip to a serving bowl.
- Serve with sliced red bell pepper strips.
- Enjoy your Greek Yogurt and Herb Dip with fresh bell pepper strips as a heart-healthy snack.

Scientific Note:

Plain Greek yogurt is an excellent source of high-quality protein and probiotics, which are beneficial for gut health. Maintaining a healthy gut can indirectly support heart health by reducing inflammation and supporting the immune system.

Dill and parsley are rich in antioxidants and provide a burst of fresh flavor without adding extra calories. These herbs have anti-inflammatory properties that support cardiovascular health. Garlic has anti-inflammatory properties and is known to support heart health by improving blood circulation and reducing blood pressure.

Lemon juice adds a refreshing flavor and is a good source of vitamin C, which has antioxidant properties that support overall health.

Olive oil is a source of healthy monounsaturated fats and omega-3 fatty acids, which help reduce inflammation and support cardiovascular health. Using olive oil instead of saturated fats can help manage cholesterol levels and improve heart function.

Red bell peppers are high in vitamins A and C, which have antioxidant properties that help protect the heart by reducing oxidative stress and inflammation. They also add a sweet and satisfying crunch to the snack.

Nutritional Information (per serving):

- Calories: ~150
- Protein: 10g
- Total Fat: 7g (mainly from olive oil and yogurt)
- Fiber: 3g
- Sodium: Low (depending on the amount of salt used)

Baked Zucchini Chips with Lemon Herb Dip

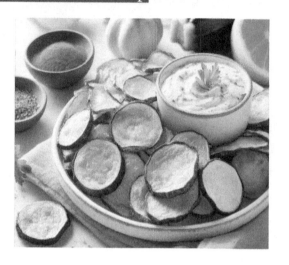

Serves: 1

Cooking Time: 25 minutes

Ingredients and Portions/Measurements:

- Zucchini (sliced into thin rounds): 1 medium (Low in calories, high in fiber, supports heart health)
- Olive Oil: 1 teaspoon (Healthy fat, supports cardiovascular health)
- Salt: A pinch (optional, use sparingly to keep sodium intake low)
- Black Pepper: A pinch (Anti-inflammatory properties)
- Garlic Powder: 1/4 teaspoon (Anti-inflammatory properties)
- Paprika: 1/4 teaspoon (Anti-inflammatory properties)

Lemon Herb Dip:

- Plain Greek Yogurt (non-fat): 1/4 cup (Rich in protein, supports heart health)
- Lemon Juice: 1 teaspoon (Adds flavor and vitamin C)
- Fresh Parsley (chopped): 1 teaspoon (Adds flavor and antioxidants)
- Salt: A pinch (optional, use sparingly to keep sodium intake low)
- Black Pepper: A pinch (Anti-inflammatory properties)

Instructions:

- Preheat the oven to 375°F (190°C).
- Place the zucchini slices in a bowl and drizzle with olive oil. Toss to coat evenly.
- Sprinkle with salt, black pepper, garlic powder, and paprika. Toss again to coat the zucchini slices evenly.
- Arrange the zucchini slices in a single layer on a baking sheet lined with parchment paper.
- Bake for 15-20 minutes, or until the zucchini slices are crispy and golden brown.
- While the zucchini chips are baking, prepare the lemon herb dip.
- In a small bowl, combine the plain Greek yogurt, lemon juice, chopped dill, chopped parsley, salt, and black pepper. Mix well until all ingredients are thoroughly combined.
- Remove the zucchini chips from the oven and let them cool slightly.
- Serve the baked zucchini chips with the lemon herb dip.
- Enjoy your Baked Zucchini Chips with Lemon Herb Dip as a heart-healthy snack.

Scientific Note:

- Zucchini is low in calories but high in essential nutrients, including vitamins A and C, which support overall health and reduce oxidative stress. It is also a good source of dietary fiber, which helps regulate cholesterol levels and supports digestive health.
- Olive oil is a source of healthy monounsaturated fats and omega-3 fatty acids, which help reduce inflammation and support cardiovascular health. Using olive oil instead of saturated fats can help manage cholesterol levels and improve heart function.
- Greek yogurt is an excellent source of high-quality protein and probiotics, which are beneficial for gut health. Maintaining a healthy gut can indirectly support heart health by reducing inflammation and

supporting the immune system.Lemon juice adds a refreshing flavor and is a good source of vitamin C, which has antioxidant properties that support overall health.

Nutritional Information (per serving):

- Calories: ~120
- Protein: 5g
- Total Fat: 7g (mainly from olive oil and yogurt)
- Fiber: 2g
- Sodium: Low (depending on the amount of salt used)

Spinach and Avocado Deviled Eggs

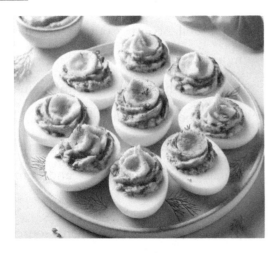

Serves: 1

Cooking Time: 20 minutes

Ingredients and Portions/Measurements:

- Large Eggs: 2 (Rich in protein, supports heart health)
- Avocado (mashed): 1/4 medium avocado (Healthy fat, contains omega-3 fatty acids, supports cardiovascular health)
- Baby Spinach (finely chopped): 1/4 cup (Packed with vitamins and minerals, supports heart health)
- Lemon Juice: 1 teaspoon (Adds flavor and vitamin C)
- Dijon Mustard: 1/2 teaspoon (Adds flavor, low in calories)
- •Salt: A pinch (optional, use sparingly to keep sodium intake low)
- Black Pepper: A pinch (Anti-inflammatory properties)
- Paprika: A pinch (Optional, for garnish)
- Fresh Dill (optional): For garnish

Instructions:

- Place the eggs in a saucepan and cover with cold water. Bring to a boil over medium-high heat. Once boiling, remove from heat, cover, and let sit for 10-12 minutes.
- Drain the hot water and transfer the eggs to an ice bath to cool. Once cooled, peel the eggs.

- Cut the eggs in half lengthwise and remove the yolks, placing them in a small bowl.
- Mash the egg yolks with the mashed avocado until smooth.
- Stir in the finely chopped spinach, lemon juice, Dijon mustard, salt, and black pepper until well combined.
- Spoon the avocado-spinach mixture back into the egg whites.
- Garnish with a pinch of paprika and fresh dill if desired.
- Serve immediately and enjoy your Spinach and Avocado Deviled Eggs as a heart-healthy snack.

Scientific Note:

Eggs are an excellent source of high-quality protein and essential amino acids, making them a heart-friendly choice for those managing AFib. They also provide important nutrients like vitamin D and choline.

Avocado is rich in monounsaturated fats, particularly omega-3 fatty acids, which help reduce inflammation and support cardiovascular health. Avocados also provide potassium, which helps regulate blood pressure—a critical factor in managing AFib.

Spinach is packed with vitamins A, C, and K, as well as minerals like magnesium and potassium, which are important for heart health. The high potassium content helps manage blood pressure, reducing the strain on the cardiovascular system.

Lemon juice adds a refreshing flavor and is a good source of vitamin C, which has antioxidant properties that support overall health.

Nutritional Information (per serving):

- Calories: ~150
- Protein: 12g
- Total Fat: 10g (mainly from eggs and avocado)
- Fiber: 2g
- Sodium: Low (depending on the amount of salt used)

Sweet Potato and Black Bean Bites

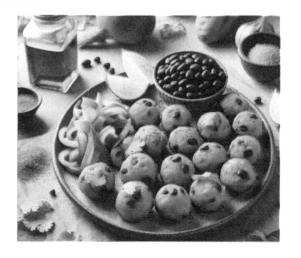

Serves: 1

Cooking Time: 30 minutes

Ingredients and Portions/Measurements:

- Sweet Potato (peeled and diced): 1 small (Rich in potassium, helps regulate blood pressure)
- Canned Black Beans (drained and rinsed): 1/4 cup (Rich in protein and fiber, supports heart health)
- Olive Oil: 1 teaspoon (Healthy fat, supports cardiovascular health)
- Red Onion (finely diced): 1 tablespoon (Anti-inflammatory properties)
- Cumin Powder: 1/2 teaspoon (Anti-inflammatory properties)
- Garlic Powder: 1/4 teaspoon (Anti-inflammatory properties)
- Salt: A pinch (optional, use sparingly to keep sodium intake low)
- Black Pepper: A pinch (Anti-inflammatory properties)
- Fresh Cilantro (chopped): 1 tablespoon (Adds flavor and antioxidants)
- Lime Wedges: For serving

Instructions:

- Preheat the oven to 375°F (190°C).
- In a bowl, combine the diced sweet potato, olive oil, cumin powder, garlic powder, salt, and black pepper. Toss to coat evenly.
- Spread the sweet potato pieces on a baking sheet lined with parchment paper and roast for 20-25 minutes until tender and lightly browned.
- In a medium-sized bowl, combine the roasted sweet potato, black beans, finely diced red onion, and chopped cilantro.
- Gently mix all the ingredients until well combined.
- Form small bite-sized balls or patties from the mixture and place them on a serving plate.
- Serve immediately with lime wedges on the side for squeezing over the bites.
- Enjoy your Sweet Potato and Black Bean Bites as a heart-healthy snack.

Scientific Note:

Sweet potatoes are rich in potassium, which helps regulate blood pressure and maintain electrolyte balance, crucial for managing AFib. They also provide dietary fiber and antioxidants, which support overall heart health.

Black beans are an excellent source of plant-based protein and dietary fiber, which help manage blood cholesterol levels and support heart health. Fiber also aids in digestion and helps maintain a healthy weight.

Red onions have anti-inflammatory properties and are known to support heart health by improving blood circulation and reducing blood pressure.

Cumin and garlic powders are spices with anti-inflammatory properties, which can help reduce inflammation and support overall heart health.

Nutritional Information (per serving):

- Calories: ~200
- Protein: 6g
- Total Fat: 5g (mainly from olive oil)
- Fiber: 6g
- Sodium: Low (depending on the amount of salt used)

Roasted Cauliflower Bites with Turmeric and Tahini Dip

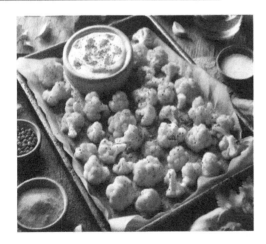

Serves: 1

Cooking Time: 25 minutes

Ingredients and Portions/Measurements:

- Cauliflower Florets: 1 cup (Rich in fiber, supports heart health)
- Olive Oil: 1 teaspoon (Healthy fat, supports cardiovascular health)
- Turmeric Powder: 1/4 teaspoon (Anti-inflammatory properties)
- Garlic Powder: 1/4 teaspoon (Anti-inflammatory properties)
- Salt: A pinch (optional, use sparingly to keep sodium intake low)
- Black Pepper: A pinch (Anti-inflammatory properties)

Tahini Dip:

- Tahini: 1 tablespoon (Rich in healthy fats, supports cardiovascular health)
- Lemon Juice: 1 teaspoon (Adds flavor and vitamin C)
- Water: 1 teaspoon (To thin the dip)
- Garlic (minced): 1/2 clove (Anti-inflammatory properties)
- Salt: A pinch (optional, use sparingly to keep sodium intake low)
- Fresh Parsley (chopped): 1 teaspoon (Adds flavour and antioxidants)

Instructions:

- Preheat the oven to 400°F (200°C).

- In a bowl, combine the cauliflower florets, olive oil, turmeric powder, garlic powder, salt, and black pepper. Toss to coat evenly.

- Spread the cauliflower florets on a baking sheet lined with parchment paper.

- Roast in the preheated oven for 20 minutes, or until the cauliflower is tender and lightly browned.

- While the cauliflower is roasting, prepare the tahini dip.

- Mix the tahini, lemon juice, water, minced garlic, salt, and chopped parsley in a small bowl until well combined.

- Remove the cauliflower from the oven and let it cool slightly.

- Serve the roasted cauliflower bites with the tahini dip.

- Enjoy your Roasted Cauliflower Bites with Turmeric and Tahini Dip as a heart-healthy snack.

Scientific Note:

- Cauliflower is low in calories but high in essential nutrients, including vitamins C and K, and fibre. It helps in reducing oxidative stress and inflammation, making it an excellent choice for heart health.

- Turmeric is known for its anti-inflammatory properties, largely due to its active compound, curcumin. It helps reduce inflammation and supports overall heart health.

- Tahini, made from sesame seeds, is rich in healthy fats, particularly omega-3 fatty acids, which help reduce inflammation and support cardiovascular health. It also provides protein and essential minerals.

Nutritional Information (per serving):

- Calories: ~150

- Protein: 5g

- Total Fat: 10g (mainly from olive oil and tahini)

- Fiber: 5g

- Sodium: Low (depending on the amount of salt used)

Edamame and Carrot Nori Rolls

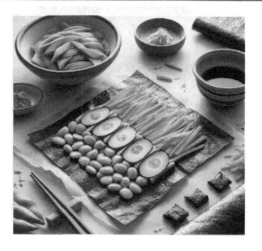

Serves: 1

Cooking Time: 15 minutes

Ingredients and Portions/Measurements:

54

- Nori Sheets: 2 (Low in calories, rich in vitamins and minerals)
- Shelled Edamame (cooked): 1/2 cup (Rich in protein and fiber, supports heart health)
- Carrot (julienned): 1 small (Rich in beta-carotene and fiber, supports overall health)
- Cucumber (julienned): 1/4 cup (Hydrating and low in calories, supports overall health)
- Avocado (sliced): 1/4 medium avocado (Healthy fat, contains omega-3 fatty acids, supports cardiovascular health)
- Brown Rice Vinegar: 1 teaspoon (Adds flavor, low in calories)
- Soy Sauce (low-sodium): 1 tablespoon (Optional, for dipping)
- Pickled Ginger (optional): For garnish

Instructions:

- Lay the nori sheets flat on a clean surface.
- In a bowl, mix the cooked edamame with brown rice vinegar.
- Spread the edamame mixture evenly over the nori sheets, leaving about an inch at the top edge.
- Layer the julienned carrot, cucumber, and avocado slices evenly over the edamame mixture.
- Carefully roll the nori sheet from the bottom edge, pressing firmly to keep the roll tight.
- Seal the edge of the nori roll with a little water.
- Cut the roll into bite-sized pieces using a sharp knife.
- Serve the nori rolls with low-sodium soy sauce for dipping and pickled ginger on the side if desired.
- Enjoy your Edamame and Carrot Nori Rolls as a heart-healthy snack.

Scientific Note:

Nori is a type of seaweed that is low in calories but rich in vitamins and minerals such as iodine, which is important for thyroid function. It also provides antioxidants that help protect the heart.

Edamame is an excellent source of plant-based protein and dietary fiber, which help manage blood cholesterol levels and support heart health. Fiber also aids in digestion and helps maintain a healthy weight, which is crucial for managing AFib.

Avocado is rich in monounsaturated fats, particularly omega-3 fatty acids, which help reduce inflammation and support cardiovascular health. Avocados also provide potassium, which helps regulate blood pressure.

Brown rice vinegar adds a tangy flavor without adding significant calories or fat, making it a great low-calorie condiment for enhancing the taste of heart-healthy snacks.

Soy sauce, when used in moderation, adds a savory flavor to the rolls. Opting for a low-sodium version helps keep sodium intake in check, which is important for managing blood pressure.

Pickled ginger adds a burst of flavor and provides antioxidants that support overall health.

Nutritional Information (per serving):

- Calories: ~180
- Protein: 8g
- Total Fat: 7g (mainly from avocado)
- Fiber: 5g
- Sodium: Low to moderate (depending on the amount of soy sauce used)
- Omega-3 Fatty Acids: ~0.5g

CONGRATULATION GOING TO DINNER RECIPES

Dear Reader,

Congratulations on completing the snacks and appetizer recipes section! I hope you found joy and deliciousness in every bite. Your culinary journey has just begun, and I'm thrilled to have you continue with us.

Your feedback is invaluable, so please leave an honest review—your thoughts will help make this book even better.

Now, let's dive into the next chapter dinner recipes. Get ready for more mouth-watering dishes that will brighten up your midday meals.

CHAPTER 5

DINNER RECIPES

Lemon Herb Salmon with Quinoa and Asparagus

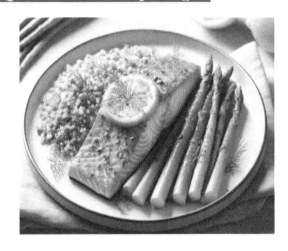

Serves: 1

Cooking Time: 25 minutes

Ingredients and Portions/Measurements:

- Salmon Fillet: 4 ounces (Rich in omega-3 fatty acids, supports cardiovascular health)
- Olive Oil: 1 teaspoon (Healthy fat, supports cardiovascular health)
- Lemon Juice: 1 tablespoon (Adds flavor and vitamin C)
- Garlic (minced): 1 clove (Anti-inflammatory properties)
- Fresh Dill (chopped): 1 tablespoon (Adds flavor and antioxidants)
- Salt: A pinch (optional, use sparingly to keep sodium intake low)
- Black Pepper: A pinch (Anti-inflammatory properties)
- Quinoa: 1/4 cup (Rich in protein, fiber, and essential amino acids; a healthy carb that's AFib friendly)
- Water: 1/2 cup (For cooking quinoa)
- Asparagus (trimmed): 6 spears (Rich in vitamins and minerals, supports heart health)

Instructions:

- Preheat the oven to 375°F (190°C).
- In a small bowl, mix the olive oil, lemon juice, minced garlic, chopped dill, salt, and black pepper.
- Place the salmon fillet on a baking sheet lined with parchment paper.
- Brush the lemon herb mixture over the salmon fillet.
- Bake in the preheated oven for 15-20 minutes, or until the salmon is opaque and flakes easily with a fork.
- While the salmon is baking, cook the quinoa: Rinse the quinoa under cold water to remove its natural coating, saponin, which can make it taste bitter or

soapy. In a small saucepan, bring water and quinoa to a boil. Reduce heat to low, cover, and simmer for 12-15 minutes or until the quinoa is tender and the water is absorbed.

- Steam the asparagus: In a steamer basket over boiling water, steam the asparagus for 5-7 minutes until tender.

- Serve the baked salmon alongside the cooked quinoa and steamed asparagus.

- Enjoy your Lemon Herb Salmon with Quinoa and Asparagus as a heart-healthy dinner.

Scientific Note:

Salmon is an excellent source of high-quality protein and omega-3 fatty acids, which are known to reduce inflammation and support cardiovascular health. Omega-3 fatty acids help lower blood pressure, reduce triglycerides, and prevent the formation of blood clots.

Quinoa is a high-quality protein that contains all nine essential amino acids. It is also rich in dietary fiber, which helps regulate cholesterol levels and supports digestive health. The fiber in quinoa also aids in maintaining a healthy weight, which is important for managing AFib.

Asparagus is low in calories and packed with essential vitamins and minerals, including vitamins A, C, E, and K, as well as folate and fiber. The antioxidants in asparagus help combat oxidative stress and inflammation, supporting overall heart health.

Nutritional Information (per serving):

- Calories: ~350

- Protein: 30g

- Total Fat: 15g (mainly from salmon and olive oil)

- Fiber: 5g

- Sodium: Low to moderate (depending on the amount of salt used)

Grilled Portobello Mushrooms with Quinoa and Roasted Veggies

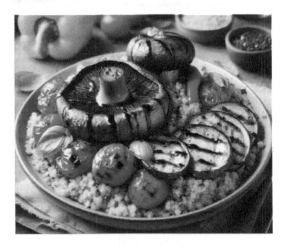

Serves: 1

Cooking Time: 30 minutes

Ingredients and Portions/Measurements:

- Portobello Mushrooms (large): 2 (Low in calories, rich in fiber, supports heart health)
- Olive Oil: 2 teaspoons (Healthy fat, supports cardiovascular health)
- Balsamic Vinegar: 1 tablespoon (Adds flavor and antioxidants)
- Garlic (minced): 2 cloves (Anti-inflammatory properties)
- Quinoa: 1/4 cup (Rich in protein, fiber, and essential amino acids; a healthy carb that's AFib friendly)
- Water: 1/2 cup (For cooking quinoa)
- Red Bell Pepper (sliced): 1/2 cup (Rich in vitamins A and C, supports heart health)
- Zucchini (sliced): 1/2 cup (Low in calories, high in fiber, supports heart health)
- Cherry Tomatoes: 1/2 cup (Rich in antioxidants, particularly lycopene, supports heart health)
- Fresh Basil (chopped): 1 tablespoon (Adds flavor and antioxidants)
- Salt: A pinch (optional, use sparingly to keep sodium intake low)
- Black Pepper: A pinch (Anti-inflammatory properties)

Instructions:

- Preheat the oven to 400°F (200°C).
- In a small bowl, mix 1 teaspoon of olive oil, balsamic vinegar, minced garlic, salt, and black pepper.
- Brush the portobello mushrooms with the balsamic mixture and let them marinate for 10 minutes.
- Place the marinated mushrooms on a baking sheet and roast for 20 minutes, or until tender.
- While the mushrooms are roasting, cook the quinoa: Rinse the quinoa under cold water to remove its natural coating, saponin, which can make it taste bitter or soapy. In a small saucepan, bring water and quinoa to a boil. Reduce heat to low, cover, and simmer for 12-15 minutes or until the quinoa is tender and the water is absorbed.
- In a separate baking dish, toss the red bell pepper, zucchini, and cherry tomatoes with the remaining olive oil, salt, and black pepper.
- Roast the vegetables in the oven for 15 minutes, or until tender and slightly caramelized.
- Remove the roasted mushrooms and vegetables from the oven.
- Serve the grilled portobello mushrooms on a plate with the cooked quinoa and roasted veggies.

- Garnish with fresh basil and enjoy your Grilled Portobello Mushrooms with Quinoa and Roasted Veggies as a heart-healthy dinner.

Scientific Note:

Portobello mushrooms are low in calories but high in essential nutrients, including vitamins and minerals that support overall health. They also provide dietary fiber, which helps regulate cholesterol levels and supports digestive health.

Quinoa is an excellent source of high-quality protein and essential amino acids, making it a heart-friendly choice for those managing AFib. It is also rich in dietary fiber, which helps regulate cholesterol levels and supports digestive health.

Red bell peppers are high in vitamins A and C, which have antioxidant properties that help protect the heart by reducing oxidative stress and inflammation. They also add a sweet and satisfying flavor to the dish.

Zucchini is low in calories and high in essential nutrients, including vitamins A and C, which support overall health and reduce oxidative stress. It is also a good source of dietary fiber, which helps regulate cholesterol levels and supports digestive health

Cherry tomatoes are rich in antioxidants, particularly lycopene, which has been shown to reduce inflammation and protect the heart. They also provide vitamins A and

C, supporting overall health and reducing oxidative stress.

Nutritional Information (per serving):

- Calories: ~300
- Protein: 10g
- Total Fat: 14g (mainly from olive oil)
- Fiber: 7g
- Sodium: Low (depending on the amount of salt used)

Herb-Crusted Cod with Spinach and Lentil Salad

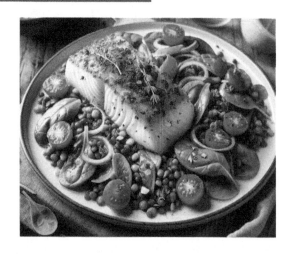

Serves: 1

Cooking Time: 30 minutes

Ingredients and Portions/Measurements:

- Cod Fillet: 4 ounces (Rich in protein, low in fat, supports heart health)
- Olive Oil: 2 teaspoons (Healthy fat, supports cardiovascular health)

60

- Fresh Parsley (chopped): 1 tablespoon (Adds flavor and antioxidants)
- Fresh Thyme (chopped): 1 teaspoon (Adds flavor and antioxidants)
- Garlic (minced): 1 clove (Anti-inflammatory properties)
- Lemon Zest: 1 teaspoon (Adds flavor and vitamin C)
- Salt: A pinch (optional, use sparingly to keep sodium intake low)
- Black Pepper: A pinch (Anti-inflammatory properties)
- Cooked Lentils: 1/2 cup (Rich in protein and fiber, supports heart health)
- Fresh Spinach: 1 cup (Packed with vitamins and minerals, supports heart health)
- Cherry Tomatoes (halved): 1/4 cup (Rich in antioxidants, particularly lycopene, supports heart health)
- Red Onion (thinly sliced): 1/4 cup (Anti-inflammatory properties)
- Balsamic Vinegar: 1 tablespoon (Adds flavor and antioxidants)

Instructions:

- Preheat the oven to 375°F (190°C).
- In a small bowl, mix 1 teaspoon of olive oil, chopped parsley, chopped thyme, minced garlic, lemon zest, salt, and black pepper.
- Brush the herb mixture over the cod fillet and place it on a baking sheet lined with parchment paper.
- Bake in the preheated oven for 15-20 minutes, or until the cod is opaque and flakes easily with a fork.
- While the cod is baking, prepare the lentil salad.
- In a medium-sized bowl, combine the cooked lentils, fresh spinach, halved cherry tomatoes, and thinly sliced red onion.
- In a small bowl, mix the remaining olive oil and balsamic vinegar. Drizzle over the lentil salad and toss to coat evenly.
- Serve the herb-crusted cod alongside the spinach and lentil salad.
- Enjoy your Herb-Crusted Cod with Spinach and Lentil Salad as a heart-healthy dinner.

Scientific Note:

Cod is a lean source of protein and provides *essential nutrients like vitamin B12 and selenium. It is low in fat and supports muscle maintenance and repair, which is important for overall health.*

Lentils are an excellent source of plant-based protein and dietary fiber, which help manage blood cholesterol levels and support heart health. Fiber also aids in digestion and helps maintain a healthy weight, which is crucial for managing AFib.

Spinach is packed with vitamins A, C, and K, as well as minerals like magnesium and potassium, which are important for heart health. The high potassium content helps manage blood pressure, reducing the strain on the cardiovascular system.

Nutritional Information (per serving):

- Calories: ~350
- Protein: 30g
- Total Fat: 10g (mainly from olive oil)
- Fiber: 8g
- Sodium: Low (depending on the amount of salt used)

Baked Lemon Garlic Chicken with Quinoa and Steamed Broccoli

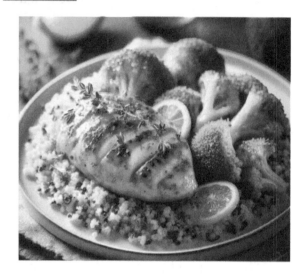

Serves: 1

Cooking Time: 30 minutes

Ingredients and Portions/Measurements:

- Chicken Breast (skinless, boneless): 4 ounces (Lean protein, supports heart health)
- Olive Oil: 2 teaspoons (Healthy fat, supports cardiovascular health)
- Lemon Juice: 2 tablespoons (Adds flavor and vitamin C)
- Garlic (minced): 2 cloves (Anti-inflammatory properties)
- Fresh Thyme (chopped): 1 teaspoon (Adds flavor and antioxidants)

- Salt: A pinch (optional, use sparingly to keep sodium intake low)
- Black Pepper: A pinch (Anti-inflammatory properties)
- Quinoa: 1/4 cup (Rich in protein, fiber, and essential amino acids; a healthy carb that's AFib friendly)
- Water: 1/2 cup (For cooking quinoa)
- Broccoli Florets: 1 cup (Rich in vitamins and minerals, supports heart health)

Instructions:

- Preheat the oven to 375°F (190°C).
- In a small bowl, mix 1 teaspoon of olive oil, lemon juice, minced garlic, chopped thyme, salt, and black pepper.
- Place the chicken breast in a baking dish and brush with the lemon garlic mixture.
- Bake in the preheated oven for 20-25 minutes, or until the chicken is cooked through and no longer pink in the center.
- While the chicken is baking, cook the quinoa: Rinse the quinoa under cold water to remove its natural coating, saponin, which can make it taste bitter or soapy. In a small saucepan, bring water and quinoa to a boil. Reduce heat to low, cover, and simmer for 12-15 minutes or until the quinoa is tender and the water is absorbed.
- Steam the broccoli: In a steamer basket over boiling water, steam the broccoli florets for 5-7 minutes until tender.
- Serve the baked lemon garlic chicken alongside the cooked quinoa and steamed broccoli.
- Enjoy your Baked Lemon Garlic Chicken with Quinoa and Steamed Broccoli as a heart-healthy dinner.

Scientific Note:

Chicken breast is a lean source of protein and provides essential nutrients like vitamin B6 and niacin. It is low in fat and supports muscle maintenance and repair, which is important for overall health.

Quinoa is an excellent source of high-quality protein and essential amino acids, making it a heart-friendly choice for those managing AFib. It is also rich in dietary fiber, which helps regulate cholesterol levels and supports digestive health.

Broccoli is packed with vitamins C and K, as well as fiber and potassium, which are important for heart health. The high fiber content helps regulate cholesterol levels and supports digestive health, while potassium helps manage blood pressure.

Nutritional Information (per serving):

- Calories: ~350
- Protein: 30g

- Total Fat: 10g (mainly from olive oil)
- Fiber: 6g
- Sodium: Low (depending on the amount of salt used)

Mediterranean Stuffed Bell Peppers

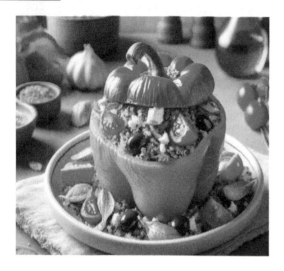

Serves: 1

Cooking Time: 40 minutes

Ingredients and Portions/Measurements:

- Bell Pepper (any color): 1 large (Rich in vitamins A and C, supports heart health)
- Quinoa: 1/4 cup (Rich in protein, fiber, and essential amino acids; a healthy carb that's AFib friendly)
- Water: 1/2 cup (For cooking quinoa)
- Olive Oil: 2 teaspoons (Healthy fat, supports cardiovascular health)
- Red Onion (diced): 1/4 cup (Anti-inflammatory properties)
- Garlic (minced): 1 clove (Anti-inflammatory properties)
- Cherry Tomatoes (halved): 1/2 cup (Rich in antioxidants, particularly lycopene, supports heart health)
- Kalamata Olives (sliced): 2 tablespoons (Optional, use sparingly for low sodium)
- Fresh Spinach (chopped): 1/2 cup (Packed with vitamins and minerals, supports heart health)
- Feta Cheese (crumbled): 2 tablespoons (Optional, for garnish, can be omitted for low sodium)
- Fresh Basil (chopped): 1 tablespoon (Adds flavor and antioxidants)
- Salt: A pinch (optional, use sparingly to keep sodium intake low)
- Black Pepper: A pinch (Anti-inflammatory properties)

Instructions:

- Preheat the oven to 375°F (190°C).
- Cut the top off the bell pepper and remove the seeds and membranes. Set aside.
- Cook the quinoa: Rinse the quinoa under cold water to remove its natural coating, saponin, which can make it taste bitter or

soapy. In a small saucepan, bring water and quinoa to a boil. Reduce heat to low, cover, and simmer for 12-15 minutes or until the quinoa is tender and the water is absorbed.

- In a medium-sized skillet, heat 1 teaspoon of olive oil over medium heat.

- Add the diced red onion and sauté for about 5 minutes until it becomes translucent.

- Add the minced garlic and cook for another 1 minute until fragrant.

- Stir in the cherry tomatoes, Kalamata olives, and chopped spinach. Cook for 3-4 minutes until the spinach is wilted and the tomatoes are slightly softened.

- Combine the cooked quinoa with the vegetable mixture and stir to combine. Season with salt and black pepper to taste.

- Stuff the bell pepper with the quinoa and vegetable mixture.

- Place the stuffed bell pepper in a baking dish and drizzle with the remaining teaspoon of olive oil.

- Bake in the preheated oven for 20-25 minutes, until the bell pepper is tender.

- Remove from the oven and sprinkle with crumbled feta cheese and chopped fresh basil.

- Serve warm and enjoy your Mediterranean Stuffed Bell Pepper as a heart-healthy dinner.

Scientific Note:

Bell peppers are high in vitamins A and C, which have antioxidant properties that help protect the heart by reducing oxidative stress and inflammation. They also add a sweet and satisfying flavor to the dish.

Quinoa is an excellent source of high-quality protein and essential amino acids, making it a heart-friendly choice for those managing AFib. It is also rich in dietary fiber, which helps regulate cholesterol levels and supports digestive health.

Spinach is packed with vitamins A, C, and K, as well as minerals like magnesium and potassium, which are important for heart health. The high potassium content helps manage blood pressure, reducing the strain on the cardiovascular system.

Cherry tomatoes are rich in antioxidants, particularly lycopene, which has been shown to reduce inflammation and protect the heart. They also provide vitamins A and C, supporting overall health and reducing oxidative stress.

Nutritional Information (per serving):

- Calories: ~300
- Protein: 10g

- Total Fat: 15g (mainly from olive oil and feta cheese)
- Fiber: 6g
- Sodium: Low to moderate (depending on the amount of salt and feta cheese used)

Sesame Ginger Tofu with Brown Rice and Steamed Bok Choy

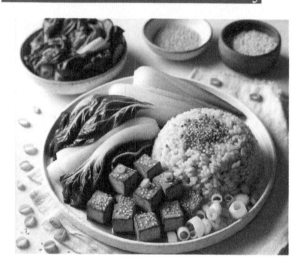

Serves: 1

Cooking Time: 30 minutes

Ingredients and Portions/Measurements:

- Firm Tofu: 4 ounces (Rich in plant-based protein, supports heart health)
- Brown Rice: 1/4 cup (Rich in fiber and essential nutrients, supports heart health)
- Water: 1/2 cup (For cooking brown rice)
- Bok Choy (sliced): 1 cup (Rich in vitamins A and C, supports heart health)
- Olive Oil: 2 teaspoons (Healthy fat, supports cardiovascular health)
- Low-Sodium Soy Sauce: 1 tablespoon (Adds flavor, low in sodium)
- Fresh Ginger (grated): 1 teaspoon (Anti-inflammatory properties)
- Garlic (minced): 1 clove (Anti-inflammatory properties)
- Sesame Seeds: 1 teaspoon (Rich in healthy fats and antioxidants)
- Green Onions (sliced): 1 tablespoon (Adds flavor and antioxidants)
- Salt: A pinch (optional, use sparingly to keep sodium intake low)
- Black Pepper: A pinch (Anti-inflammatory properties)

Instructions:

- Cook the brown rice: Rinse the brown rice under cold water. In a small saucepan, bring water and brown rice to a boil. Reduce heat to low, cover, and simmer for 25-30 minutes or until the rice is tender and the water is absorbed.
- While the rice is cooking, prepare the tofu: Press the tofu to remove excess moisture, then cut into cubes.
- In a medium-sized skillet, heat 1 teaspoon of olive oil over medium heat. Add the

tofu cubes and cook until golden brown on all sides, about 8-10 minutes.

- In a small bowl, mix the low-sodium soy sauce, grated ginger, and minced garlic. Pour over the tofu and cook for another 2-3 minutes until the tofu is well coated and heated through.
- Steam the bok choy: In a steamer basket over boiling water, steam the bok choy for 5-7 minutes until tender.
- Assemble the dish: Serve the cooked tofu over the brown rice and steamed bok choy.
- Garnish with sesame seeds and sliced green onions.
- Enjoy your Sesame Ginger Tofu with Brown Rice and Steamed Bok Choy as a heart-healthy dinner.

Scientific Note:

Tofu is a rich source of plant-based protein and provides essential amino acids. It is low in saturated fat and supports muscle maintenance and repair, which is important for overall health.

Brown rice is an excellent source of dietary fiber, which helps regulate cholesterol levels and supports digestive health. The fiber in brown rice also aids in maintaining a healthy weight, which is important for managing AFib.

Bok choy is packed with vitamins A, C, and K, as well as minerals like calcium and potassium, which are important for heart health. The high potassium content helps manage blood pressure, reducing the strain on the cardiovascular system.

Nutritional Information (per serving):

- Calories: ~300
- Protein: 15g
- Total Fat: 10g (mainly from olive oil and sesame seeds)
- Fiber: 6g
- Sodium: Low to moderate (depending on the amount of soy sauce used)

Lemon Herb Chicken with Wild Rice and Steamed Green Beans

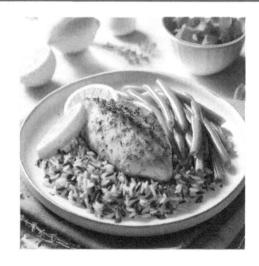

Serves: 1

Cooking Time: 35 minutes

Ingredients and Portions/Measurements:

- **Chicken Breast (skinless, boneless):** 4 ounces (Lean protein, supports heart health)
- **Olive Oil:** 2 teaspoons (Healthy fat, supports cardiovascular health)
- **Lemon Juice:** 2 tablespoons (Adds flavor and vitamin C)
- **Garlic (minced):** 2 cloves (Anti-inflammatory properties)
- **Fresh Thyme (chopped):** 1 teaspoon (Adds flavor and antioxidants)
- **Salt:** A pinch (optional, use sparingly to keep sodium intake low)
- **Black Pepper:** A pinch (Anti-inflammatory properties)
- **Wild Rice:** 1/4 cup (Rich in fiber and essential nutrients, supports heart health)
- **Water:** 1/2 cup (For cooking wild rice)
- **Green Beans:** 1 cup (Rich in vitamins and minerals, supports heart health)

Instructions:

- Preheat the oven to 375°F (190°C).
- In a small bowl, mix 1 teaspoon of olive oil, lemon juice, minced garlic, chopped thyme, salt, and black pepper.
- Place the chicken breast in a baking dish and brush with the lemon herb mixture.
- Bake in the preheated oven for 25-30 minutes, or until the chicken is cooked through and no longer pink in the center.
- While the chicken is baking, cook the wild rice: Rinse the wild rice under cold water. In a small saucepan, bring water and wild rice to a boil. Reduce heat to low, cover, and simmer for 25-30 minutes or until the rice is tender and the water is absorbed.
- Steam the green beans: In a steamer basket over boiling water, steam the green beans for 5-7 minutes until tender.
- Serve the lemon herb chicken alongside the cooked wild rice and steamed green beans.
- Enjoy your Lemon Herb Chicken with Wild Rice and Steamed Green Beans as a heart-healthy dinner.

Scientific Note:

Chicken breast is a lean source of protein and provides essential nutrients like vitamin B6 and niacin. It is low in fat and supports muscle maintenance and repair, which is important for overall health.

Wild rice is an excellent source of dietary fiber, which helps regulate cholesterol levels and supports digestive health. The fiber in wild rice also aids in maintaining a healthy weight, which is important for managing AFib.

Green beans are packed with vitamins A, C, and K, as well as fiber and potassium, which are important for heart health. The high fiber content helps regulate cholesterol levels and supports digestive health, while potassium helps manage blood pressure.

Nutritional Information (per serving):

- Calories: ~350
- Protein: 30g
- Total Fat: 10g (mainly from olive oil)
- Fiber: 6g
- Sodium: Low (depending on the amount of salt used)

Turmeric Ginger Baked Salmon with Sweet Potato Mash and Steamed Asparagus

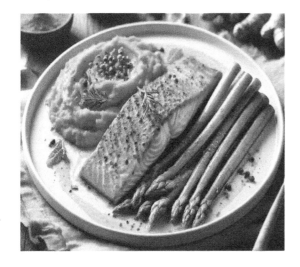

Serves: 1

Cooking Time: 30 minutes

Ingredients and Portions/Measurements:

- **Salmon Fillet:** 4 ounces (Rich in omega-3 fatty acids, supports cardiovascular health)
- **Olive Oil:** 2 teaspoons (Healthy fat, supports cardiovascular health)
- **Turmeric Powder:** 1/2 teaspoon (Anti-inflammatory properties)
- **Fresh Ginger (grated):** 1 teaspoon (Anti-inflammatory properties)
- **Garlic (minced):** 1 clove (Anti-inflammatory properties)
- **Salt:** A pinch (optional, use sparingly to keep sodium intake low)
- **Black Pepper:** A pinch (Anti-inflammatory properties)
- **Sweet Potato (peeled and diced):** 1 medium (Rich in potassium and fiber, supports heart health)
- **Low-Sodium Vegetable Broth:** 1/4 cup (For cooking sweet potato)
- **Asparagus (trimmed):** 1 cup (Rich in vitamins and minerals, supports heart health)

Instructions:

- Preheat the oven to 375°F (190°C).
- In a small bowl, mix 1 teaspoon of olive oil, turmeric powder, grated ginger, minced garlic, salt, and black pepper.

- Place the salmon fillet on a baking sheet lined with parchment paper. Brush with the turmeric ginger mixture.
- Bake in the preheated oven for 15-20 minutes, or until the salmon is opaque and flakes easily with a fork.
- While the salmon is baking, cook the sweet potato: In a medium saucepan, add the diced sweet potato and vegetable broth. Bring to a boil, then reduce heat and simmer until the sweet potato is tender, about 10-15 minutes.
- Mash the cooked sweet potato until smooth. Add a pinch of salt and black pepper to taste.
- Steam the asparagus: In a steamer basket over boiling water, steam the asparagus for 5-7 minutes until tender.
- Serve the baked salmon alongside the sweet potato mash and steamed asparagus.
- Enjoy your Turmeric Ginger Baked Salmon with Sweet Potato Mash and Steamed Asparagus as a heart-healthy dinner.

Scientific Note:

Salmon is an excellent source of high-quality protein and omega-3 fatty acids, which are known to reduce inflammation and support cardiovascular health. Omega-3 fatty acids help lower blood pressure, reduce triglycerides, and prevent the formation of blood clots.

Sweet potatoes are rich in potassium, which helps regulate blood pressure and maintain electrolyte balance, crucial for managing AFib. They also provide dietary fiber and antioxidants, which support overall heart health.

Asparagus is packed with vitamins A, C, and K, as well as fiber and potassium, which are important for heart health. The high fiber content helps regulate cholesterol levels and supports digestive health, while potassium

Nutritional Information (per serving):

- Calories: ~350
- Protein: 25g
- Total Fat: 15g (mainly from salmon and olive oil)
- Fiber: 6g
- Sodium: Low (depending on the amount of salt used)

Balsamic Glazed Turkey Meatballs with Quinoa and Roasted Brussels Sprouts

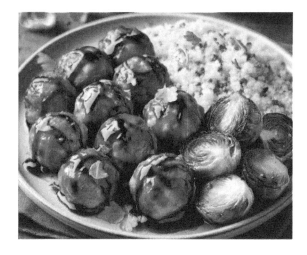

Serves: 1

Cooking Time: 35 minutes

Ingredients and Portions/Measurements:

- **Ground Turkey (lean):** 4 ounces (Lean protein, supports heart health)
- **Quinoa:** 1/4 cup (Rich in protein, fiber, and essential amino acids; a healthy carb that's AFib friendly)
- **Water:** 1/2 cup (For cooking quinoa)
- **Brussels Sprouts (halved):** 1 cup (Rich in vitamins and minerals, supports heart health)
- **Olive Oil:** 2 teaspoons (Healthy fat, supports cardiovascular health)
- **Balsamic Vinegar:** 2 tablespoons (Adds flavor and antioxidants)
- **Garlic (minced):** 1 clove (Anti-inflammatory properties)
- **Fresh Parsley (chopped):** 1 tablespoon (Adds flavor and antioxidants)
- **Salt:** A pinch (optional, use sparingly to keep sodium intake low)
- **Black Pepper:** A pinch (Anti-inflammatory properties)

Instructions:

- Preheat the oven to 375°F (190°C).
- In a small bowl, mix 1 teaspoon of olive oil, balsamic vinegar, minced garlic, salt, and black pepper.
- In a medium bowl, combine the ground turkey, chopped parsley, and half of the balsamic mixture. Form the mixture into small meatballs.
- Place the meatballs on a baking sheet lined with parchment paper and bake for 20-25 minutes, or until the meatballs are cooked through and no longer pink in the center.
- While the meatballs are baking, prepare the quinoa: Rinse the quinoa under cold water. In a small saucepan, bring water and quinoa to a boil. Reduce heat to low, cover, and simmer for 12-15 minutes or

until the quinoa is tender and the water is absorbed.

- In a medium bowl, toss the halved Brussels sprouts with the remaining teaspoon of olive oil, salt, and black pepper.

- Spread the Brussels sprouts on a separate baking sheet and roast in the oven for 15-20 minutes, or until tender and slightly caramelized.

- Remove the meatballs and Brussels sprouts from the oven.

- Serve the turkey meatballs with the cooked quinoa and roasted Brussels sprouts. Drizzle the remaining balsamic mixture over the meatballs.

- Enjoy your Balsamic Glazed Turkey Meatballs with Quinoa and Roasted Brussels Sprouts as a heart-healthy dinner.

Scientific Note:

Ground turkey is a lean source of protein and provides essential nutrients like vitamin B6 and niacin. It is low in fat and supports muscle maintenance and repair, which is important for overall health.

Quinoa is an excellent source of high-quality protein and essential amino acids, making it a heart-friendly choice for those managing AFib. It is also rich in dietary fiber, which helps regulate cholesterol levels and supports digestive health.

Brussels sprouts are packed with vitamins C and K, as well as fiber and antioxidants, which are important for heart health. The high fiber content helps regulate cholesterol levels and supports digestive health, while antioxidants help reduce oxidative stress.

Nutritional Information (per serving):

- Calories: ~350

- Protein: 30g

- Total Fat: 12g (mainly from olive oil and turkey)

- Fiber: 7g

- Sodium: Low to moderate (depending on the amount of salt used)

CHAPTER 6

14 DAYS MEAL PLAN

Day 1

Breakfast: Berry Quinoa Breakfast Bowl (7:00 AM)

Lunch: Grilled Chicken and Quinoa Salad (12:00 PM)

Snack: Avocado and Edamame Dip with Veggie Sticks (3:00 PM)

Dinner: Lemon Herb Salmon with Quinoa and Asparagus (7:00 PM)

Day 2

Breakfast: Blueberry Chia Pudding (7:00 AM)

Lunch: Lentil and Vegetable Soup (12:00 PM)

Snack: Cucumber and Hummus Bites (3:00 PM)

Dinner: Grilled Portobello Mushrooms with Quinoa and Roasted Veggies (7:00 PM)

Day 3

Breakfast: Spinach and Tomato Egg White Omelette (7:00 AM)

Lunch: Chickpea and Spinach Stew (12:00 PM)

Snack: Roasted Red Pepper and Chickpea Mini Wraps (3:00 PM)

Dinner: Herb-Crusted Cod with Spinach and Lentil Salad (7:00 PM)

Day 4

Breakfast: Greek Yogurt Parfait with Flaxseed and Berries (7:00 AM)

Lunch: Mediterranean Stuffed Bell Peppers (12:00 PM)

Snack: Greek Yogurt and Herb Dip with Bell Pepper Strips (3:00 PM)

Dinner: Baked Lemon Garlic Chicken with Quinoa and Steamed Broccoli (7:00 PM)

Day 5

Breakfast: Apple Cinnamon Overnight Oats (7:00 AM)

Lunch: Grilled Salmon with Mango Avocado Salsa (12:00 PM)

Snack: Baked Zucchini Chips with Lemon Herb Dip (3:00 PM)

Dinner: Mediterranean Stuffed Bell Peppers (7:00 PM)

Day 6

Breakfast: Smoked Salmon and Avocado Toast (7:00 AM)

Lunch: Zucchini Noodles with Pesto and Cherry Tomatoes (12:00 PM)

Snack: Spinach and Avocado Deviled Eggs (3:00 PM)

Dinner: Sesame Ginger Tofu with Brown Rice and Steamed Bok Choy (7:00 PM)

Day 7

Breakfast: Spinach and Mushroom Egg White Scramble (7:00 AM)

Lunch: Sweet Potato and Black Bean Taco (12:00 PM)

Snack: Sweet Potato and Black Bean Bites (3:00 PM)

Dinner: Lemon Herb Chicken with Wild Rice and Steamed Green Beans (7:00 PM)

Day 8

Breakfast: Tropical Smoothie Bowl (7:00 AM)

Lunch: Chickpea and Spinach Stuffed Portobello Mushrooms (12:00 PM)

Snack: Roasted Cauliflower Bites with Turmeric and Tahini Dip (3:00 PM)

Dinner: Turmeric Ginger Baked Salmon with Sweet Potato Mash and Steamed Asparagus (7:00 PM)

Day 9

Breakfast: Apple and Almond Butter Breakfast Wrap (7:00 AM)

Lunch: Lemon Herb Quinoa Salad with Grilled Shrimp (12:00 PM)

Snack: Edamame and Carrot Nori Rolls (3:00 PM)

Dinner: Balsamic Glazed Turkey Meatballs with Quinoa and Roasted Brussels Sprouts (7:00 PM)

Day 10

Breakfast: Berry Quinoa Breakfast Bowl (7:00 AM)

Lunch: Grilled Chicken and Quinoa Salad (12:00 PM)

Snack: Avocado and Edamame Dip with Veggie Sticks (3:00 PM)

Dinner: Moroccan Chickpea Stew with Couscous (7:00 PM)

Day 11

Breakfast: Blueberry Chia Pudding (7:00 AM)

Lunch: Lentil and Vegetable Soup (12:00 PM)

Snack: Cucumber and Hummus Bites (3:00 PM)

Dinner: Herb-Crusted Cod with Spinach and Lentil Salad (7:00 PM)

Day 12

Breakfast: Spinach and Tomato Egg White Omelette (7:00 AM)

Lunch: Chickpea and Spinach Stew (12:00 PM)

Snack: Roasted Red Pepper and Chickpea Mini Wraps (3:00 PM)

Dinner: Baked Lemon Garlic Chicken with Quinoa and Steamed Broccoli (7:00 PM)

Day 13

Breakfast: Greek Yogurt Parfait with Flaxseed and Berries (7:00 AM)

Lunch: Mediterranean Stuffed Bell Peppers (12:00 PM)
Snack: Greek Yogurt and Herb Dip with Bell Pepper Strips (3:00 PM)
Dinner: Lemon Herb Salmon with Quinoa and Asparagus (7:00 PM)

Snack: Baked Zucchini Chips with Lemon Herb Dip (3:00 PM)
Dinner: Grilled Portobello Mushrooms with Quinoa and Roasted Veggies (7:00 PM)

Day 14

Breakfast: Apple Cinnamon Overnight Oats (7:00 AM)
Lunch: Grilled Salmon with Mango Avocado Salsa (12:00 PM)

ASKING FOR YOUR HONEST REVIEW

Dear Reader,

Thank you for taking the time to read my cookbook. I hope you found the recipes delightful and that they added a special touch to your meals. Your feedback is incredibly valuable to me, as it helps me improve and continue sharing delicious recipes with you.

If you enjoyed the book, or if you have any suggestions for improvement, I would be grateful if you could leave an honest review. Your thoughts and experiences are important, and they will also help other readers in making informed decisions.

Thank you once again for your support and for being a part of this culinary journey with me

2 WEEKS MEAL PLANNER

WEEKLY MEAL PLANNER __1__

MONDAY

BREAKFAST _____

LUNCH _____

SNACKS _____

DINNER _____

TUESDAY

BREAKFAST _____

LUNCH _____

SNACKS _____

DINNER _____

WEDNESDAY

BREAKFAST _____

LUNCH _____

SNACKS _____

DINNER _____

THURSDAY

BREAKFAST _____

LUNCH _____

SNACKS _____

DINNER _____

FRIDAY

BREAKFAST _____

LUNCH _____

SNACKS _____

DINNER _____

SATURDAY

BREAKFAST _____

LUNCH _____

SNACKS _____

DINNER _____

SUNDAY

BREAKFAST _____

LUNCH _____

SNACKS _____

DINNER _____

NOTES

_____

_____

_____

_____

WEEKLY MEAL PLANNER __2__

MONDAY

BREAKFAST _____

LUNCH _____

SNACKS _____

DINNER _____

TUESDAY

BREAKFAST _____

LUNCH _____

SNACKS _____

DINNER _____

WEDNESDAY

BREAKFAST _____

LUNCH _____

SNACKS _____

DINNER _____

THURSDAY

BREAKFAST _____

LUNCH _____

SNACKS _____

DINNER _____

FRIDAY

BREAKFAST _____

LUNCH _____

SNACKS _____

DINNER _____

SATURDAY

BREAKFAST _____

LUNCH _____

SNACKS _____

DINNER _____

SUNDAY

BREAKFAST _____

LUNCH _____

SNACKS _____

DINNER _____

NOTES

_____

_____

_____

_____

Made in the USA
Las Vegas, NV
09 October 2024

96536242R00044